ACUTE REVASCULARIZATION OF THE INFARCTED HEART

ACUTE REVASCULARIZATION OF THE INFARCTED HEART

A Society of Cardiovascular Anesthesiologists Monograph

Edited by

J. G. Reves, M.D.

Professor of Anesthesiology
Duke University Medical Center
Durham, North Carolina

Grune & Stratton, Inc.
Harcourt Brace Jovanovich, Publishers
Orlando   New York   San Diego   London
San Francisco   Tokyo   Sydney   Toronto

Grune & Stratton, Inc.
Orlando, Florida 32887

Distributed in the United Kingdom by
Grune & Stratton, Ltd.
24/28 Oval Road, London NW 1

Library of Congress Catalog Number 87-80331
International Standard Book Number 0-8089-1870-2
Printed in the United States of America
87 88 89 90   10 9 8 7 6 5 4 3 2 1

Publication Committee of the
Society of Cardiovascular Anesthesiologists

Norig Ellison, M.D.
Judith A. Fabian, M.D.
David Gaba, M.D.
Simon Gelman, M.D.
Mark Hilberman, M.D.
Tricia Kapur, M.D.
Robert A. Kates, M.D.
J. G. Reves, M.D.
Steve Tosone, M.D.

CONTENTS

Foreword   IX
Preface   XIII
Contributors   XVII

Chapter 1. The Scientific Foundations for
Reperfusion of the Acutely
Ischemic Myocardium   1
John H. Tinker

Chapter 2. The Management of Acute
Myocardial Infarction Using
Thrombolysis and Emergency
Angioplasty   17
Richard S. Stack

Chapter 3. Reperfusion of the Acute
Myocardial Infarction: Role of
Anesthesia   35
*Robert A. Kates, Russell Hill, and
J. G. Reves*

Chapter 4. Intervention in Acute Myocardial
Infarction: The Role of Surgical
Management   65
*Robert A. Guyton, David A.
Langford, Joseph M. Arcidi, Jr.,
Douglas C. Morris, Henry A.
Liberman, and Charles R. Hatcher Jr.*

Index   85

FOREWORD

Coronary artery disease leading to acute myocardial infarction continues to be the major health problem for Western civilization. Revascularization of the heart during the course of acute myocardial infarction has the potential to be the most important therapeutic modality yet devised. The role of reperfusion currently is undergoing extensive clinical investigation. In this monograph the initial paper by Dr. J. H. Tinker defines much of the current scientific rationale underlying revascularization as a method of achieving myocardial salvage. The next three papers detail techniques employed to achieve coronary reperfusion. These papers cover the field clearly and there is little need for me to be redundant. Thus I will not provide a brief synopsis of these papers in this foreword. Instead, I would like to present my perspectives concerning the potential benefits to be derived from reperfusing the ischemic heart of patients with acute myocardial infarction.

I would like to advance the proposal that the major goal of reperfusion is to affect in a positive way both the long-term survival of the patient and to maximize myocardial function. At first it would seem obvious that these goals are achieved by limiting the degree of myocardial necrosis. Thus, the principles outlined in Dr. Tinker's paper are of paramount importance i.e., reperfusion must be accomplished early enough to salvage a significant amount of myocardium. This will in turn result in improvement in both ventricular function and survival. This reasoning suggests that if reperfusion does not take place early enough to salvage significant myocardial tissue, then no benefit will result.

The major question is whether the only factor involved is the magnitude of myocardial salvage. There are at least some data that would indicate that other factors may be involved. In an earlier study Shaw et al[1] noted that apical venting of patients undergoing bypass surgery resulted in apical dyskinesia or akinesia in 56 percent whereas only 8 percent of the patients with mitral stenosis who underwent valvulotomy through a dilator inserted into the apex of the left ventricle had dyskinesia. These investigators postulated that the perfusion of the area of the ventriculotomy was better in the latter group, which resulted in better healing and consequently reduced the incidence of apical dysfunction. The hypothesis to be advanced from these data is that given an area of irreversibly injured myocardium the healing process may be positively affected by reperfusion leading to less thinning of the myocardium and better scar formation.

The prognosis in the acute phase of myocardial infarction has been demonstrated clearly to be improved by reperfusion.[2] However, the long-term effects of reperfusion on outcome are still somewhat in doubt, although initial data indicate that the long-term prognosis also will be considerably improved if vessel patency is maintained. Recently, Stadius et al[3] showed that complete reperfusion during acute myocardial infarction is associated with a higher probability of survival at one year for any particular ejection fraction than would be expected with conservative therapy. During the past 10 years 103 patients undergoing bypass surgery at Duke Medical Center had a concomitant acute myocardial infarction during the procedure with persistent new Q waves indicating significant myocardial necrosis. Following discharge the one-year survival in this group of patients was 95 percent. Although the data are not strictly comparable, of the 2250 patients surviving a myocardial infarction and treated without reperfusion who were discharged from Duke Hospital from 1969 to 1983, the one year survival was 84 percent. Although the two groups are not strictly comparable in a variety of factors, including the degree of ventricular dysfunction, these data strongly suggest that patients with myocardial infarction occurring during the trauma of bypass surgery have a lower long-term fatality rate. The earlier and more complete Q-wave resolution that we have observed in these patients compared to medically treated patients implies that reperfusion with bypass grafting has resulted in a different process of "infarct healing."

Several mechanisms may be operative in improving the prognosis following reperfusion when the affected vessel remains patent. As noted above, reperfusion may enhance the healing process. In addition a widely patent coronary artery may reduce future episodes of reocclusion. In the case of multivessel disease the patent artery may provide blood to collateral vessels in the event that another large coronary artery acutely occludes. Finally, reperfusion potentially may reduce the instance of fatal arrhythmias. Thus it seems that the hypothesis that survival may be enhanced by reperfusion regardless of the degree of myocardial salvage is not only tenable but entirely reasonable.

Clearly we have the available expertise and methodology to reperfuse the ischemic myocardium in a large proportion of patients suffering acute myocardial infarction. My guess is that this therapy will significantly improve the longterm survival of patients even in the absence of demonstrable initial myocardial salvage.

BIBLIOGRAPHY

1. Shaw RA, Kong Y, Pritchett ELC, et al: Ventricular apical vents and postoperative focal contraction abnormalities in patients undergoing coronary artery bypass surgery. Circulation 55:434–438, 1977
2. Gruppo Italiano Per Lo Studio Della Streptochinasi Nell'Infarto Miocardico (GISSI): Effectiveness of intravenous thrombolytic treatment in acute myocardial infarction. Lancet 397–401, 1986
3. Stadius ML, Davids K, Maynard C, et al: Risk stratification for 1 year survival based on characteristics identified in the early hours of acute myocardial infarction. Circulation 74:703–711, 1986

Joseph C. Greenfield, Jr., M.D.
Professor and Chairman
Department of Internal Medicine
Duke University Medical Center
Durham, North Carolina

PREFACE

Acute Revascularization of the Infarcted Heart is the inaugural monograph in a series of annual volumes sponsored by the Society of Cardiovascular Anesthesia. The Society was founded in 1978 with the primary purpose of educating physicians interested in cardiovascular medicine, surgery, and anesthesia. Annual scientific meetings and workshops have achieved this purpose. Annual meetings have limitations, however, since most of the content is in oral form and not all members of the Society or others interested in the proceedings are able to attend. Thus, the Board of Directors created a publication committee to determine if the Society should publish scientific material to achieve the educational goals of the Society.

The publication committee studied a number of publication formats and objectives—always with the knowledge that there is a wealth of written information available to members of the Society. The proposal that the Society sponsor a scientific journal was fully explored and decided against.

The concept of an annual monograph was the product of two ideas. First, the annual meeting was very successful and always covered at least one important and timely topic. Secondly, an educational benefit for *all* members of the Society would enhance the value of the Society to its members. Thus, the concept of an annual monograph emanating from the annual meeting and distributed to all Society members was proposed to the publication committee and adopted by the board in 1985.

An annual monograph will be published each year by the Society and distributed to all members of the Society as a membership benefit. The volume is published by Grune & Stratton and through their offices and agents the book will be offered for sale to the entire medical community. Each monograph is devoted entirely to one of the topics addressed at the annual meeting of the Society of Cardiovascular anesthesiologists. The written word becomes a permanent record of one topic at the annual meeting; however, by design the monograph is more comprehensive than the lecture. Only timely authoritative reviews will be published in the monograph series.

As with any sponsored monograph, legitimate questions arise concerning peer review and whether the book officially represents the Society, its collective members, or its officers. Peer review is assured by having each of the manuscripts reviewed by the editor and at least one member of the publication committee. This is not as rigorous peer review as some publications, but there is a mechanism to reject an unacceptable manuscript. Also, relatively uniform style can be achieved. The Society does not endorse the contents of the monograph as policy or as a reflection of the opinion of the members and officers. The monograph does reflect the considered views of each author and as such is a worthwhile contribution to the education of the Society membership.

The topic of the annual monograph is chosen by the publication committee and the annual meeting program committee. Once the topic is decided then the moderator of the meeting panel is chosen and asked to serve as the editor. These decisions are made in consultation with the program and publication committees. The editor chooses the contributing participants, and may solicit supplemental contributions and contributors to fully cover the subject. Each monograph will cover topics selected because of its relevance and timeliness. Monographs are to be concise yet definitive. Some will be longer than others depending on complexity of the topic.

Acute Revascularization of the Infarcted Heart has chapters from three medical centers, where contributors are all active in the clinical care and research of the field. Joseph C. Greenfield, Jr., M.D., Professor and Chairman of Internal Medicine at Duke University Medical Center authored the foreword. Dr. Greenfield is a cardiologist, researcher, and scholar in the field of cardiovascular medicine. In his foreword, he perfectly places this topic in the overall management of ischemic heart disease. The reason to revascularize the infarcted heart is to "effect in a positive way both the long-term survival of the patient and to maximize myocardial function." He advances the intriguing notion that even without short-term functional improvement aggressive early revascularization will extend life. We will have to await long-term results of these procedures to see if Dr. Greenfield is correct.

Dr. John Tinker is Professor and Chairman of the Department of Anesthesiology at the University of Iowa. Dr. Tinker has had a productive research career in cardiovascular anesthesiology, and his chapter reviews the available literature and animal experimentation supporting the concept of acute reperfusion of the ischemic and infarcted heart. The concept of optimal time of reperfusion is advanced as well as controversies regarding the clinical revascularization.

Richard Stack, M.D., is the director of the Duke University interventional cardiac medicine program. He and his colleagues have pioneered the various medical strategies now used in effecting reperfusion of the infarcted heart. He discusses thrombolytic and angioplasty treatment modalities and reports the clinical results from Duke.

Three members of the division of cardiothoracic anesthesia at Duke, Rob Kates, M.D., Russell Hill, M.D., and the editor presented the evidence for the hypothesis that anesthesia protects the ischemic or jeopardized heart. Pertinent review of the literature of anesthetics on myocardial salvage as well as results of two clinical studies are reported. Problems of anesthetic management for patients with acute infarction are presented as well as some possible solutions.

R. A. Guyton, M.D., and his surgical associates present the rationale for surgical reperfusion of the ischemic and infarcted heart. The Emory University surgical results are placed in perspective of other centers and treatment modalities.

This monograph is incomplete. A more detailed discussion of thrombolytic therapy or discussion of reperfusion arrhythmias would have broadened the subject. Certainly proof that acute reperfusion is beneficial would be welcome, especially considering that all the strategies discussed in this book require 24 hours a day commitments of highly skilled, well trained professionals. The interventional management is more expensive than simple intensive care "wait and see" approaches. However, if this book does nothing more, it demonstrates that acute reperfusion of the infarcted heart can be safely accomplished, and asks the ultimate question does acute revascularization extend life?

It is my hope that this first Society monograph is helpful to the Society and to others who read it. If it does contribute to our education in a useful way, then the many who have had part in its making will be gratified.

CONTRIBUTORS

Joseph M. Arcidi, Jr., M.D. *Departments of Surgery and Medicine, The Carlyle Fraser Heart Center, Crawford W. Long Memorial Hospital, Emory University School of Medicine, Atlanta, Georgia*

Robert A. Guyton, M.D. *Departments of Surgery and Medicine, The Carlyle Fraser Heart Center, Crawford W. Long Memorial Hospital, Emory University School of Medicine, Atlanta, Georgia*

Charles R. Hatcher, Jr., M.D. *Department of Surgery and Medicine, The Carlyle Fraser Heart Center, Crawford W. Long Memorial Hospital, Emory University School of Medicine, Atlanta, Georgia*

Russell Hill, M.D. *Duke University Medical Center, Durham, North Carolina*

Robert A. Kates, M.D. *Duke University Medical Center, Durham, North Carolina*

David A. Langford, M.D. *Departments of Surgery and Medicine, The Carlyle Fraser Heart Center, Crawford W. Long Memorial Hospital, Emory University School of Medicine, Atlanta, Georgia*

Henry A. Liberman, M.D. *Departments of Surgery and Medicine, The Carlyle Fraser Heart Center, Crawford W. Long Memorial Hospital, Emory University School of Medicine, Atlanta, Georgia*

Douglas C. Morris, M.D. *Departments of Surgery and Medicine, The Carlyle Fraser Heart Center, Crawford W. Long Memorial Hospital, Emory University School of Medicine, Atlanta, Georgia*

J. G. Reves, M.D. *Professor of Anesthesiology, Duke University Medical Center, Durham, North Carolina*

Richard S. Stack, M.D., F.A.C.C. *Director, Intervention Cardiac Catheterization Program, Duke University Medical Center, Durham, North Carolina*

John H. Tinker, M.D. *Professor and Head, Department of Anesthesia, University of Iowa, Iowa City, Iowa*

ACUTE REVASCULARIZATION OF THE INFARCTED HEART

The Scientific Foundations for Reperfusion of the Acutely Ischemic Myocardium

John H. Tinker

One can legitimately ask "is there, in fact, any scientific foundation for attempting, by any means, to reperfuse acutely ischemic
myocardium?" Are the changes toward cell death so rapid as to
render attempts at reperfusion futile? Are there really such things
as "golden periods" or "border zones," implying potentially
(partially) successful reperfusion?

Braunwald,[1] in a recent perspective on the subject, states "not
since Herrick's original description of acute myocardial infarction
(AMI) have so many options been available for the treatment of
this condition." Clearly all that was available until recently was
bed rest, oxygen, and attempts at prevention of the usual complications of bed rest. The near universal acceptance of coronary care
units implied to the public that specific therapy existed, but
actually they were little more than intensive vigilance areas,
monitoring for arrhythmias and attempting rapid responses to
them. Despite these modalities AMI remains the most common
cause of *in-hospital* death in industrialized nations!

ACUTE REVASCULARIZATION OF THE INFARCTED HEART   ISBN 0-8089-1870-2
Copyright © 1987 by Grune & Stratton, Inc.   All rights reserved.

1

Morbidity of survivors of AMI is another crucial issue. It is clear that this morbidity is markedly dependent upon degree of dysfunction of the left ventricle. The latter is largely dependent on the sizes of the original infarction plus any "aftershocks," i.e., myocardium which becomes infarcted later.

There are, again according to Braunwald,[1] two other corollary areas of concern. Obviously there is a time limit in each patient beyond which potential salvage approaches a vanishing point. A 4-hour figure is often quoted as this magic number, but it must vary greatly depending on many individual factors. For example, if the initial area of ischemia is large, then the resultant demands placed on the remaining functional myocardium will be proportionally great. Border zones surrounding the infarcting area might therefore get less oxygen delivery than if the original infarct was smaller, thus the larger the initial infarct, the more likely additional myocardium is to be drawn into it. Many other factors, especially collateralization, play roles as well. Therefore, timelines on intervention must be understood and must be capable of occurring on a nationwide basis, not just in sophisticated tertiary care centers, if acute therapy for AMI is to succeed in its twin goals of limiting the original infarction and preventing additional tissue death.

Much of the basic research in this area has been performed in animal models, especially the dog. In this monograph, we will try to delineate and summarize that research to see if there is in fact much of a scientific basis for believing that we can, given current options, be successful in achieving prevention of mortality, limitation of infarct size, and subsequent amelioration of morbidity, and prevention of "aftershocks" or additional infarctions occurring as a direct result of the original AMI.

CAN (SHOULD) MYOCARDIUM BE "SALVAGED"?

If you occlude a major coronary artery in a dog, approximately 20 percent of the animals will die within the first half hour. These animals have generally been considered to be analogous to those humans who succumb to arrhythmias during the early period (sometimes seconds or minutes) following AMI—the group for which coronary care units, EKG telemetered ambulances etc., were evolved. If the artery is left occluded for 1–2 hours in the dog and then released, there will be a smaller resultant infarct than if the artery was permanently occluded. After 4–6 hours of occlusion, if the ligature is released, the immediate death rate will be higher, and the resultant infarct will often be *larger* than in the animals with permanent occlusions. In the reperfused group (after 4–6 hours' occlusion) intramyocardial hemorrhage can often be seen, presumably due to breakdown of capillary integrity in the infarcted zone.[2–3]

The issue gets much more complicated. Extent of infarction may very well depend upon how it is measured. For example, if wall motion studies are used in vivo during AMI, even for several days after AMI, larger areas of infarction may be noted than can actually be confirmed later histologically. This discrepancy gave rise to the concept that some myocardial tissue may be "stunned" during AMI, i.e., dysfunctional but salvaged somehow and eventually able to return to functionality.[4–7] This helps explain why there are all sorts of discrepancies in the literature as to the "effects" of various "treatments" during AMI. Salvaged myocardium may be truly salvaged, in the sense that it can return to full function, or it may remain somewhat contractile but certainly not fully functional (the term "dysfunctional" is very inadequate to describe this tissue). Ellis et al[8] attempted to quantitate the relation between actual transmural extent of AMI and *eventual* associated regional contractility patterns in dogs after left anterior descending coronary artery (LAD) ligation. They studied permanent occlusion versus 2-hour occlusions. They compared two dimensional echocardiographic computer assisted regional wall motion analyses with eventual histologic infarct localization by triphenyl tetrazolum chloride (TTC) staining technique (both of these widely used for purposes of quantitating functional versus histologic aspects of AMI). They compared noninfarcted regions with those containing infarct with respect to wall thickening (function). In noninfarct containing regions, the wall thickened 59 ± 16 percent during contractions. In infarct-containing regions, the LV wall thickened minus 4–47 percent, depending to some degree on how much histologic infarct was present in the region studied.[8] The reason for going into detail about this particular study is to emphasize the complexity of studying myocardial salvage. In the Ellis et al study, there was a reasonable correlation (−87 percent) between degree of regional function (measured by wall thickening) and percentage of that region histologically infarcted.[8]

Most clinical trials which have attempted to measure salvage have not reported much, if any, recovery of overall left ventricular ejection fraction after reperfusion. Two such studies, the Western Washington Intracoronary Streptokinase trial[9] and the European Registry,[10] found increases in ejection fraction compared to controls (during AMI) of 0 and 5 percent, respectively, when patients were studied 4 weeks or more after AMI. This result might have indicated little salvage, or it might merely have reflected compensation by surrounding well perfused myocardium during the AMI (controls).[8] Ellis et al[8] suggest that an additional explanation might be that "[resultant] function may not be linearly related to the amount of salvage and that salvage of small amounts of myocardium is of little functional consequence." Indeed, when less than 40 percent of an expected resultant infarct was salvaged, in the Ellis et al[8] dog study, there was little benefit with respect to subsequent overall myocardial function.

Therefore, the issue of salvage and how to measure its functional consequences is by far the most central issue with respect to development of an adequate experimental model. The issue of when to perform intervention is less interesting, since clinically, physicians are likely to try to perform whatever intervention is in vogue just as soon as practicable during AMI anyway.

Hammerman et al[11] studied dogs using 2-D echo versus eventual histologic outcome. The dogs had 6-hour coronary occlusions, or two-hour occlusions followed by 4-hour reperfusions. The resultant mass of necrosis was 74 percent of the area at risk when a 6-hour occlusion was used versus 44 percent when a 2-hour occlusion plus 4 hours of reperfusion was studied. Despite this obvious eventual salvage, 2-D echocardiographic wall motion studies could not detect it—i.e., wall motion abnormalities were of similar extent in the two groups. Their contention is that it might not be prudent to conclude, based on in vivo wall motion studies in humans, that particular interventions were ineffective.[11] Intuitively it seems logical that if well perfused myocardium can compensate during AMI by increasing its contractility, then overall indices of function, especially ejection fraction, might be maintained throughout AMI (in survivors). If so, then myocardium which actually was salvaged by some intervention or other might go undetected. Thus it might not be reasonable to conclude, as have several authors,[1,9,10] that various interventions do not help salvage myocardium. Is it worth salvaging these smaller amounts of tissue? Those who glibly state that there is no superfluous myocardium might be reminded of the morbidity and mortality rates associated with all the interventions proposed to date. We just do not have the answers at this time.

Therefore, there are two sides to the salvage question. Side one says that you can salvage smaller masses of myocardial tissue and yet not detect the resultant salvage by global or even regional functional means, and therefore you should persist with therapy. Side two says that if the global function is not likely to be improved by such "small" (less than 40 percent of expected infarct) salvage, then maybe it is not worth the morbidity/mortality price which must be paid during and following the interventions.

Nuclear magnetic resonance (NMR) has been used in a canine model to study another aspect of reperfusion, namely edema formation.[12] Brown et al[12] found that acute ischemia of at least 1 hour in duration resulted in detectable myocardial edema which can be followed with several NMR evaluations. Their contention was that perhaps this newer method would allow use of edema regression rates as evidence for salvage.

Various forms of computed tomography have also been used to study the reperfusion versus salvage question. For example, Mancini et al,[13] again using dogs, studied permanent versus 2-hour occlusions followed by unlimited reperfusion. They followed the animals for several days. Both groups experienced severe early changes, but the permanently occluded group remained severely depressed with respect to regional wall thickening 3 days later whereas the reperfused group, despite equally severe initial wall motion depression, experienced some improvement at 3 days. The wall thickening in the ischemic zone of the nonreperfused animals was about 2 percent at 3 days versus 17 percent at 3 days for the reperfused animals. Despite this average "improvement," these changes were not statistically significant. Again, as noted above, despite not being able to convincingly document salvage by reperfusion after 2 hours' occlusion using in vivo techniques, there was a clear salvage histologically.[13]

Summarizing the salvage question, the literature regarding whether or not a new drug, operation, or angioplasty has resulted in actual salvage must very much depend on: (1) how salvage was measured; (2) how salvage was determined; (3) whether salvage was determined using indices of global or regional LV function; (4) whether there were any histologic correlations; and (5) whether the actual salvage resulted in worthwhile improvement in subsequent expectable myocardial function and/or quality of life, especially compared with the mortality/morbidity prices paid during the salvaging intervention(s).

WHAT ABOUT COLLATERALS? DOGS VERSUS PIGS? HUMANS?

The dog has a relatively well but variably collateralized myocardial circulation. It is possible to occlude a major coronary artery in a dog and not produce any resultant infarct. If radioactive microspheres are injected into the coronary artery just prior to its occlusion at the same location, subsequent autoradiographic techniques can easily determine the area "at risk," i.e., where the microspheres lodged. After the AMI is developed (6 hours to 2 days), TTC staining will reveal the actual resultant infarct. In normal dogs, the infarct size, taken as a percent of the original area at risk, is depressingly variable (ranging from 0 to 75 percent!). This calls dog studies of salvage after reperfusion into question if the controls were other dogs wherein the coronary artery was permanently ligated. If, on the other hand, the dog is used (as reported above) in studies looking to assess in vivo versus histologic evaluations of resultant infarct, there is validity.

Some contend that because the dog is a collateralized animal, it may be a suitable analog with respect to comparisons to collateralized humans, namely humans with relatively longstanding coronary artery disease. The trouble with that idea is that dogs' collaterals are not developed in response to disease. Indeed, dogs left to their own devices do not die of coronary artery disease (perhaps their lives are not "stressful" enough). Humans, before their first MI and before long years of periodic angina pectoris, do not have well collateralized myocardia. Therefore, at the very least, the dog would not seem to be a particularly good model to study humans who have not yet had reasons to develop collaterals.

Pigs, however, are so "noncollateralized" that 75–90 percent of the area "at risk," determined as above, will infarct after permanent occlusion. Further, upon TTC staining, the infarcts appear much more homogeneous than do those in dogs. Indeed the pig would possibly die of coronary artery disease (except that pigs grow so large and unwieldly that there have not been good studies!). With such an end-arterial coronary circulation, the pig would be likely to receive much more new blood flow during reperfusion to a region of myocardium beyond a previous ligature than would the dog, if the collaterals in the dog had been supplying at least some blood to the region during the period of occlusion. Thus, although there is little evidence, reperfusion might be more beneficial with respect to salvage of tissue in the pig than in the dog. The point of this discussion is not to extol the virtues of pigs over dogs in this kind of research, but rather to make the point that value of reperfusion with respect to salvage of myocardium may well depend upon degree of collateralization previously present.

Presently, we have little knowledge of how collaterals develop in response to coronary artery disease, whether we can predict their existence in a given patient, and how to study their function. Blanke et al[14] chose to replace the term collaterals with residual flow to the infarct zone. They studied the latter by coronary angiography in 130 patients during AMI. In 36 patients the artery supplying the AMI zone was incompletely obstructed, i.e., there was "residual antegrade flow" to the infarct zone. In 56 patients there was complete inflow obstruction but there was residual flow, presumably via collaterals, into the infarct zone. In the remaining 38 patients, with AMI, there was neither antegrade nor collateral flow observable into the zone of infarction. Ejection fractions during AMI averaged, interestingly, 55, 48, and 50 percent respectively and, although the group with remaining antegrade flow had statistically better LV EF, these 3 averages are convincing that global indices are of relatively little value in assessing eventual salvage or efficacy of therapy. The patients in whom there was observable collateral flow into the zone of AMI had a longer history of angina pectoris.[14]

Of the 130 patients in the study by Blanke et al,[14] 37 did not undergo any reperfusion therapy. They did, however, have repeat angiography later. Ejection fractions did not change between the acute and chronic stages of infarction (either way—up or down) if there was observable antegrade flow originally during the AMI. The patients who had observable collateral flow into the AMI also did not deteriorate chronically with respect to LV EF. The patients who had no observable antegrade or collateral flow into the AMI *did* undergo significant worsening of ejection fraction (a *further* average decrease of 10 percent). These authors contend, therefore, with excellent human evidence, that presence of collateral flow into an AMI, versus absence of same, probably is a very important determinant of whether any reperfusion intervention will have a demonstrable efficacy, at least with respect to global post infarction function.[14] It is logical that the patient having an early AMI, who has *not* had previous MIs, who has *not* had a long (or any) history of angina pectoris, might *not* be expected to have much collateral ("residual") flow into the infarct zone. These patients might superficially be expected to benefit most from reperfusion. Analyzing this question a bit further however leads to the speculation that these patients might be just the ones in whom the golden period would be the shortest. These are the patients who would have to be treated earliest if significant myocardial salvage was to be achieved. Further, it is just such patients in whom denial of developing AMI might be expected to delay therapy the longest—since those patients would not be as likely to understand what was occuring. This, again, points out the complexities associated with the simple starting idea of attempting reperfusion during AMI. Other authors[15–20] are in substantial agreement with the findings of Blanke et al[14] and the above analysis.

ARE THERE OTHER FACTORS THAT MIGHT DETERMINE OUTCOME/ADVISABILITY OF REPERFUSION DURING AMI?

Sheehan et al[21] studied 47 patients with AMI who underwent reperfusion (proven angiographically) after streptokinase therapy. Their endpoint was recovery of LV function after perfusion. They avoided the global compensation problems mentioned above by measuring regional LV function via ventriculography. An important determinant of functional improvement was, logically, diameter of the resultant stenosis after reperfusion was achieved. This is often ignored, perhaps as being too simple, but lysis of the thrombus "straw that broke the camel's back" still leaves the patient with a residual stenosis. Sheehan et al clearly showed that LV functional outcome was partly dependent upon the size of this critical residual stenosis.[21] Mere achievement of angiographic evidence that *some* flow is now getting past a previously (presumably acutely) obstructed area clearly takes a lower priority to achievement of adequate flow.[21] The Sheehan et al[21] study also showed that patients in whom angiographic reperfusion was achieved within 2 hours of onset of symptoms had better resultant regional myocardial function than those in whom reperfusion was achieved but not until after 2 hours.[21] Marx et al[22] also showed that adequate flow, not just angiographic evidence of reperfusion, is essential and that severe residual stenosis prevented same. Harrison et al[23] reported the greater risk of rethrombosis and further AMI when residual stenosis was severe. There is not universal agreement on this point. Smalling et al[24] could not correlate functional outcome with residual percent (estimated) stenosis. Sheehan et al[21] point out that merely thinking of residual stenosis in terms of percentage occlusion may be insufficient. The actual shape of the cross section at the point of stenosis may be a critically important determinant of what happens next at that point after reperfusion has been achieved.[21]

Unlike the series of Blanke et al,[14] wherein about one third of the patients had observable collaterals, Sheehan et al reported that only 3 (6 percent) of their patients had collaterals. Perhaps the better functional result achieved in the Sheehan et al[21] study was due to selection of patients *without* demonstrable collaterals.

Mathey et al[25] reported that if reperfusion could be achieved within 2 hours of onset of symptoms, wall motion resulting at chronic follow-up was near normal in 82 percent of patients (14 of 17 patients), whereas if reperfusion was achieved 2–5 hours after symptom onset wall motion was improved toward normal in only 46 percent (24 of 52 patients). The relative sizes of populations here is interesting, because it indicates that in only 17 of 69 patients, for whatever reason, could reperfusion be achieved within 2 hours of onset of symptoms. As noted by Braunwald,[1] it is unlikely that anywhere near this percentage of Americans undergoing AMI could be treated with any remotely complex form of therapy within 2 hours of onset of symptoms.

Wei et al[26] studied another aspect of the reperfusion question, namely reflexes which might be stimulated by achievement of reperfusion. In a group of 41 AMI patients, 27 had "successful" reperfusions. Of those, 17 developed major bradycardia and hypotension, while 1 other patient developed tachycardia and hypertension all at the approximate time of achievement of recanalization. They concluded that "successful" reperfusion seems to stimulate the cardioinhibitory vasodepressor ("Bezold-Jarish") reflexes. Whether this could be used to predict spontaneous occurrence of reperfusion is unknown.[26,27] This does, however, bring up a very important aspect of the discussion of evaluation of success, or salvage or function. Ejection fraction is well known to be a markedly rate-dependent measure. If "control" versus "post reperfusion" versus "chronic" ejection fractions were not performed at similar heart rates, then results are open to question. Clearly reflex vasodilation and/or bradycardia are well known to be associated with coronary angiography.[28–30]

Ganz[31] reported that reperfusion was heralded in many patients with arrhythmias, some life threatening. This, again, brings up the point that if a significant number of patients are lost due to the reperfusion, whether by iatrogenic complications related to the treatment or to arrhythmias possibly resulting from reperfusion itself, then these "costs" must be quantitated against the salvage benefits.

ARE THERE DIFFERENCES IN METHODOLOGY VERSUS OUTCOME?

This is the subject of several other monographs. Suffice it to say here that streptokinase,[19,32,33] given via the intracornary or intravenous routes, urokinase,[34] intracoronary beta adrenergic blockade,[35] acute balloon angioplasty,[36–38] acutely performed coronary bypass,[39–41] bypass after streptokinase, digitalis plus one or more of the above,[42] converting enzyme inhibitors,[43] new beta blockers like exaprolol,[44] the alpha adrenergic antagonist nicergaline,[45] naloxone for arrythmias,[46] and various antiinflammatory drugs,[47] have all been reported, often in combination with other therapies. We are probably not far enough along to be able to determine a treatment of choice because we still are unsure about how to actually determine salvage and/or the functional result of same.

SUMMARY AND CONCLUSIONS

If you acutely occlude a coronary artery, in dog, pig, or man, and release the occlusion after a few seconds, you get an infarction. As you approach 20 minutes, depending on many factors, there will be damage. As you approach 4–6 hours, there will be a point at which release of the ligature will not have measurable benefit. In man, the "golden period" is probably 2 hours, with perhaps an additional "silver" period (my term) of another 2–3 hours wherein some benefit may be achieved. In any event, there is presumably a period during which reperfusion will be of benefit in each patient.

How much benefit will accrue is dependent upon many factors including: size of the residual stenosis; presence or absence of collateral inflow to the ischemic zone; whether abnormal reflexes and/or arrhythmias occurred with the intervention; and presumably what other morbidity might have occurred associated with or as a result of the intervention.

Students of the question of efficacy of reperfusion must examine in detail the salvage question, for if the endpoint is to be measurable functional improvement (global), then the results achieved with reperfusion are nowhere near as encouraging as those achieved when the endpoint is either regional functional improvement or actual histologic salvage. Still, the latter two methods do make sense. It is logical that more tissue alive and functioning would be likely (except possibly for arrhythmias) to result in better physiologic quality of life however difficult that is to measure.

My answer to the question "Is there a scientific foundation to the concept that reperfusion is a worthwhile therapeutic goal?" is a very heavily qualified "yes," given the provisos detailed above.

REFERENCES

1. Braunwald E: The aggressive treatment of acute myocardial infarction. Circulation 71:1087–1092, 1985

2. Maroko PR, Libby P, Ginks WR, et al: Coronary artery reperfusion I. Early effects on local myocardial function and the extent of myocardial necrosis. J Clin Invest 51:2710–2716, 1972

3. Reimer KA, Lowe JE, Rasmussen MM, et al: The wave front phenomenon of myocardial ischemic death I. Myocardial infarct size versus duration of coronary occlusion in dogs. Circulation 56:786–794, 1977

4. Roan PE, Scales F, Saffer F, et al: Functional characterization of left ventricular segmental responses during the initial 24 hour and 1 week after experimental canine myocardial infarction. J Clin Invest 64:1074–1088, 1979

5. Lieberman AN, Weiss JL, Jugdutt BI, et al: Two dimensional echocardiography and infarct size: relationship of regional wall motion and thickening to the extent of myocardial infarction in the dog. Circulation 63:739–746, 1981

6. Theroux P, Ross J, Franklin D, et al: Regional myocardial function and dimensions early and late after myocardial infarction in the unanesthetized dog. Circ Res 40:158–165, 1977

7. Ellis SG, Henschke CI, Sandor T, et al: Time course of functional and biochemical recovery of myocardium salvaged by reperfusion. J Am Coll Cardiol 1:1047–1055, 1983

8. Ellis SG, Henschke CI, Sandor T, et al: Relation between the transmural extent of acute myocardial infarction and associated myocardial contractility two weeks after infarction. Am J Cardiol 55:1412–1416, 1985

9. Kennedy JW, Ritchie JL, Davies KB, et al: Western Washington randomized trial intracoronary streptokinase in acute myocardial infarction. N Engl J Med 309:1477–1482, 1983

10. Rentrop P, Smith H, Painter L, et al: Changes in left ventricular ejection fraction after intracoronary thrombolytic therapy. Circulation (suppl.) 1:55–60, 1983

11. Hammerman H, O'Boyle JE, Cohen C, et al: Dissociation between two dimensional echocardiographic left ventricular wall motion and myocardial salvage in early experimental acute myocardial infarction in dogs. Am J Cardiol 54:875–879, 1984

12. Brown JJ, Strich G, Higgins CB, et al: Nuclear magnetic resonance analysis of acute myocardial infarction in dogs: the effect of transient coronary ischemia of varying duration in reperfusion on spin lattice relaxation times. Am Heart J 109:486–490, 1985

13. Mancini GBJ, Peck WW, Slutksy RA, et al: Use of computerized tomography to assess myocardial infarct size in ventricular function in dogs during acute coronary occlusion and reperfusion. Am J Cardiol 53:282–289, 1984

14. Blanke H, Cohen M, Karsch KR, et al: Prevalence and significance of residual flow to the infarct zone during the acute phase of myocardial infarction. J Am Coll Cardiol 5:827–831, 1985

15. Rogers WJ, Hood WP, Mantle JA, et al: Return of left ventricular function after reperfusion in patients with myocardial infarction: importance of subtotal stenosis or intact collaterals. Circulation 69:338–339, 1984

16. Nohara R, Kambara H, Murakami T, et al: Collateral function in early acute myocardial infarction. Am J Cardiol 52:955–959, 1983

17. Fulton WFM: The time factor in the enlargement of an anastomoses in coronary artery disease. Scot Med J 9:18–23, 1964

18. Khouri EM, Gregg DE, McGranahan GM: Regression and reappearance of coronary collaterals. Am J Physiol 220:655–661, 1971

19. Rentrop P, Cohen M, Phillips R, et al: Acute changes in collateral filling during transluminal coronary angioplasty. Eur Heart J 5(suppl. I):i–110, 1984

20. Mathey DG, Kuck KH, Tilsner V, et al: Non-surgical coronary artery recanalization in acute transmural myocardial infarction. Circulation 63:489–497, 1981

21. Sheehan FH, Mathey DG, Schofer J, et al: Factors that determine recovery of left ventricular function after thrombolysis in patients with acute myocardial infarction. Circulation 71:1121–1128, 1985

22. Marx W, Bethge C, Effert S, et al: Supraselective fibrinolysis and acute myocardial infarction. Bibl Haematol 47:205, 1981

23. Harrison DG, Ferguson DW, Collins SM, et al: Rethrombosis after reperfusion with streptokinase: importance of geometry of residual lesions. Circulation 69:991, 1984

24. Smalling RW, Fuentes F, Matthews MW, et al: Sustained improvement in left ventricular function in mortality by intracoronary streptokinase administration during evolving myocardial infarction. Circulation 68:131, 1983

25. Mathey DG, Sheehan FH, Schofer J, et al: Time from onset of symptoms to thromboblytic therapy: a major determinant of myocardial salvage in patients with acute transmural infarction. J Am Coll Cardiol 6:518–525, 1985

26. Wei JY, Markis JE, Malagold M, et al: Cardiovascular reflexes stimulated by reperfusion of ischemic myocardium and acute myocardial infarction. Circulation 67:796–801, 1983

27. Ong L, Reiser P, Coromilas J, et al: Left ventricular function and

rapid release of creatine kinase MB in acute myocardial infarction: evidence for spontaneous reperfusion. N Engl J Med 309:1–6, 1983

28. Eckberg DL, White CW, Kioschos JM, et al: Mechanisms mediating by the cardia during coronary arteriography. J Clin Invest 54:1455, 1974

29. Zelis R, Caudill CC, Baggett K, et al: Reflex vasodilation induced by coronary angiography in human subjects. Circulation 53:490, 1976

30. Perez-Gomez F, Garcia-Aguado A: Origin of ventricular reflexes caused by coronary arteriography. Br Heart J 39:967, 1977

31. Ganz W: Intracoronary thrombolysis in acute myocardial infarction. Am J Cardiol 52(suppl. I):92a–95a, 1983

32. Leiboff RH, Katz RJ, Wasserman AG, et al: A randomized, angiographically controlled trial of intracoronary streptokinase in acute myocardial infarction. Am J Cardiol 53:404–407, 1984

33. Golf SW, Temme H, Kempf KD, et al: Systemic short-term fibrinolysis with high-dose streptokinase in acute myocardial infarction: time course of biochemical parameters. J Clin Chem Clin Biochem 22:723–729, 1984

34. Mathey DG, Schofer J, Sheehan FH, et al: Intravenous urokinase in acute myocardial infarction. Am J Cardiol 55:878–882, 1985

35. Gold HJ, Leinbach RC, Harper RW: Usefulness of intravenous propranolol in predicting left anterior descending blood flow during anterior myocardial infarction. Am J Cardiol 54:264–268, 1984

36. Pepine CJ, Prida X, Hill JA: Percutaneous transluminal coronary angioplasty in acute myocardial infarction. Am Heart J 107:820–822, 1984

37. Holmes DR, Smith HC, Vilestra RE, et al: Percutaneous transluminal coronary angioplasty, alone or in combination with streptokinase therapy during acute myocardial infarction. Proc Mayo Clin 60:449–456, 1985

38. Hartzler GO, Rutherford BD, McConahay DR: Percutaneous transluminal coronary angioplasty: application for acute myocardial infarction. Am J Cardiol 53:117C–121C, 1984

39. Silverman NA: The surgeons role in the treatment of acute myocardial infarction. Surg Clin North Am 65:527, 1985

40. DeWood MA, Spores J, Berg R, et al: Acute myocardial infarction: a decade of experience with surgical reperfusion in 701 patients. Circulation 68(suppl. II):II-8–II-16, 1983

41. Losman JG, Finchum RN, Nagle D, et al: Myocardial surgical revascularization after streptokinase treatment for acute myocardial infarction. J Thorac Cardiovasc Surg 89:24–34, 1985

42. Bigger JT, Fleiss JL, Rolnitzky LM, et al: Effective digitalis treatment

on survival after acute myocardial infarction. Am J Cardiol 55:623–630, 1985

43. Hock CE, Ribiero LGT, Lefer AM: Preservation of ischemic myocardium by a new converting enzyme inhibitor, enalaprilic acid, in acute myocardial infarction. Am Heart J 109:222–228, 1985

44. Parratt JR, Udvary E: The effect of exaprolol (MG 8823) on epicardial ST segment changes in a feline model of acute myocardial ischaemia. Br J Pharmac 80:95–105, 1983

45. Bolli R, Brandon TA, Fisher DJ, et al: Beneficial effects of alpha-adrenergic antagonist nicergoline during acute myocardial ischemia and reperfusion in the dog. Am Heart J 106:1014–1023, 1983

46. Bergy JL, Beil ME: Anti-arrhythmic evaluation of naloxone against acute coronary occlusion—induced arrhymias in pigs. Eur J Pharmacol 90:427–431, 1983

47. Mullane KM, Read N, Salmon JA, et al: Role of leukocytes in acute myocardial infarction in anesthetized dogs: relationship to myocardial salvage by anti-inflammatory drugs. J Pharmacol Exp Ther 228:510–522, 1984

The Management of Acute Myocardial Infarction Using Thrombolysis and Emergency Angioplasty

Richard S. Stack

Death due to cardiovascular disease continues to be the number one cause of mortality in the United States. In 1985, there were over one million patients who suffered acute myocardial infarction. Five-hundred fifty thousand of these patients died as a result. Recently, however, it has become clear that early and aggressive management of acute myocardial infarction can significantly reduce both the morbidity and mortality of this disease.

EXPERIMENTAL STUDIES OF MYOCARDIAL SALVAGE

Early studies in animals showed that reperfusion following periods of up to 6 hours of temporary occlusion resulted in histologic evidence of myocardial salvage. Reimer et al showed that significant salvage of myocardium was time-dependent, but could occur after several hours of temporary occlusion in the dog.[1,2] Figure 2-1 shows that histologic evidence of myocardial

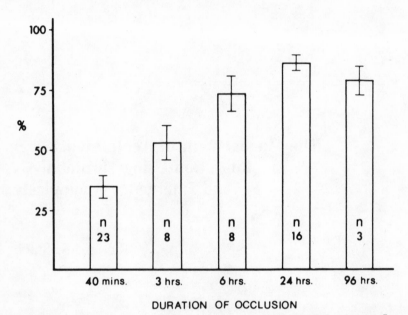

DURATION OF OCCLUSION

Fig. 2-1. Percent of myocardium in the distribution of the circumflex coronary artery showing histologic evidence of necrosis following temporary coronary occlusion ranging from 40 minutes to 96 hours in 58 dogs. (Reprinted from Reimer K, Lowe J, Rasmussen M, et al: Myocardial infarct size versus duration of coronary occlusion in dogs. Circulation 56:786–794, 1977. Reprinted by permission of the American Heart Association.)

salvage fell off rapidly and was essentially absent after 6 hours of temporary occlusion. Theroux et al showed that reperfusion after 2 hours of temporary coronary occlusion in dogs resulted in a delayed functional improvement in the center and particularly at the margins of the jeopardized region of myocardium 2–4 weeks after the ischemic event.[3] Puri et al found a 60 percent improvement in segmental wall motion at 2 weeks following a 3-hour period of temporary coronary occlusion.[4]

CLINICAL STUDIES OF CORONARY REPERFUSION

Initial studies of functional salvage in man using the global ejection fraction showed little improvement among patients treated with intracoronary streptokinase compared to controls.[5–7]

ACUTE   CHRONIC

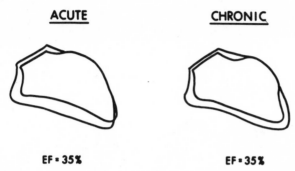

EF = 35%   EF = 35%

Fig. 2-2. Tracing on the left shows a ventricular silhouette in the right anterior oblique projection obtained during the acute study. The tracing on the right is in the same projection at the time of hospital discharge showing improvement in the region of the jeopardized myocardium, normalization of the initial hyperdynamic segments in the compensatory region, and no change in the global ejection fraction measurement.

In an early study from our laboratory, however, we theorized that these findings could result from hyperdynamic compensatory changes in the uninvolved segments of myocardium during the initial ventriculographic study compared to the ventriculogram taken prior to hospital discharge.[8] This concept is illustrated in Figure 2-2. The ventriculogram obtained during the acute cardiac catheterization showed akinesia in the region of the jeopardized myocardium. In order to maintain cardiac output there was a significant increase in sympathetic tone during the first several hours of cardiac injury. This resulted in a marked hyperdynamic compensatory wall motion of the uninvolved segments of the myocardium. In this example, at the time of hospital discharge there was a 50 percent improvement in regional wall motion in the region of the infarct following successful reperfusion. Despite this major salvage of jeopardized myocardium, the overall global ejection fraction showed no change since the improvement in function in the jeopardized region now allowed the hyperdynamic compensatory region to return to normal while still maintaining an adequate cardiac output. The regional wall motion analysis from this study is summarized in Figures 2-3 and 2-4. Patients

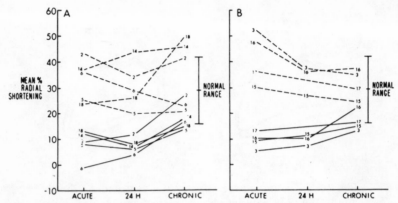

Fig. 2-3. (A) Percent radial shortening (RS) in all patients with acute and chronic catheterization studies who were initially reperfused and who showed a significant (≥5 percent) improvement in angiographic EF between the acute and chronic study. Changes in the percentage RS in the jeopardized region are shown using solid lines while changes in the compensatory region are shown using interrupted lines. The normal range (mean ± 2SD) for percentage RS in 58 normal patients is shown on the right. (B) Percentage RS in patients with acute and chronic catheterization studies who were initially reperfused and who showed no change or a decrease in the EF between the acute and chronic studies. (Reprinted from Stack RS, Phillips HR, Grierson DS, et al: Functional Improvement of Jeopardized Myocardium Following Intracoronary Streptokinase Infusion in Acute Myocardial Infarction. J Clin Invest. 72:84, 1983. With permission.)

who had greater than 5 percent improvement in global ejection fraction at the time of discharge are shown in Figure 1-3, Panel A. Each patient demonstrated improvement in the region of the jeopardized myocardium often into the low normal range. Similarly, patients who showed *no change or a decrease* in their overall ejection fraction (Fig. 2-3, Panel B) also showed uniform improvement in the region of the jeopardized myocardium. Thus, the fall in ejection fraction was caused by relaxation of the initially hyperdynamic compensatory wall motion in the *uninvolved* segments in each case. Patients who could not be reperfused (Fig. 1-4), however, showed no change or a decrease in the function of the jeopardized region as well as the overall global

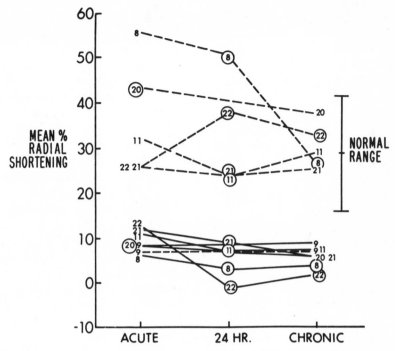

Fig. 2-4. Percentage RS in all patients with acute and chronic catheterization studies who were not reperfused during the acute study or who later reoccluded after initial recanalization. A circle around the patient number indicates that the infarct-related vessel was open at the end of that study. Changes in the percentage RS in the jeopardized region are shown using solid lines while changes in the compensatory region are shown using interrupted lines. (Reprinted from Stack RS, Phillips HR, Grierson DS, et al: Functional Improvement of Jeopardized Myocardium Following Intracoronary Streptokinase Infusion in Acute Myocardial Infarction. J Clin Invest. 72:84, 1983. With permission.)

ejection fraction in each case. It is interesting to note that patients who were open at the time of the 24-hour study (Fig. 2-4, open circles) but who were not reperfused at the time of the initial study also showed no improvement in regional or global left ventricular function at the time of the late (predischarge) study.

While this investigation demonstrated salvage of function

following reperfusion of ischemic myocardium in man, there were two major limitations: (1) the overall success rate for effective recanalization using intracoronary streptokinase alone was only 63 percent and (2) in patients who were successfully reperfused, there was a significant residual narrowing remaining at the site of previous obstruction in each patient. The mean residual luminal diameter narrowing among patients successfully reperfused was 85 percent. Thus, the residual stenosis was not unlike the preinfarct state of the plaque. Consequently, in this group of patients, there was a 30 percent incidence of reinfarction during the subsequent hospitalization.

Despite the demonstration of salvage of myocardial function after successful reperfusion, several small studies designed to compare survival among patients treated with streptokinase compared to placebo showed conflicting results.[9-11] Each of these studies, however, were characterized by a sample size that was too small to detect a significant difference in mortality. Recently, several large randomized studies have shown a significant improvement in survival among patients treated with streptokinase compared to placebo controls.[12-14] The Gruppo Italiano Per Lo Studio Della Streptochinasi Nell'Infarto Miocardico (GISSI) Study, which randomized 11,806 patients, showed a 47 percent improvement in survival in patients treated with intravenous streptokinase during the first hour after myocardial infarction.[14] The improvement in survival was time dependent, however, and was not significant if streptokinase was administered more than 6 hours after the onset of chest pain.

DUKE EXPERIENCE USING EMERGENCY PERCUTANEOUS TRANSLUMINAL CORONARY ANGIOPLASTY: THE INTERVENTIONAL CARDIAC CATHETERIZATION PROGRAM

Because of the limitations of thrombolytic therapy alone, we hypothesized that the immediate use of percutaneous transluminal coronary angioplasty (PTCA) during acute infarct could improve the initial success rate and reduce the residual coronary stenosis. The use of PTCA during acute myocardial infarction was

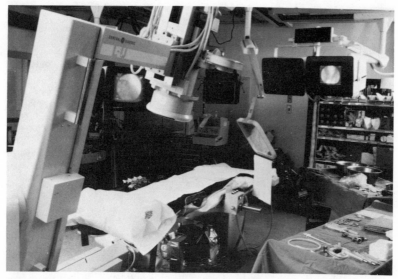

Fig. 2-5. View of the Interventional Cardiac Catheterization Laboratory showing the large screen high resolution monitors (above, left) and digital playback monitors (above, right).

first reported by Meyer et al[15] in 1982. Since that time, only a small number of studies with limited numbers of patients have been reported. In order to test this approach in a large scale clinical trial, Duke established a committed Interventional Cardiac Catheterization (ICC) Program specializing in the management of acute myocardial infarction with PTCA. A specialized ICC Laboratory, devoted exclusively to PTCA, was built adjacent to the Emergency Room. A helicopter transport system was established to service referring hospitals within 150 miles of Duke. The laboratory was equipped with large screen, high resolution video fluoroscopy and digital arteriographic equipment to allow immediate decisions regarding the nature of the coronary lesion and PTCA outcome without the usual delays associated with processing cine film (see Figs. 2-5 and 2-6). A three bed holding unit was built in the Emergency Room and three helipads were constructed near the Emergency Room entrance. The laboratory was staffed with 2 senior staff, 1 cardiology fellow, and 4

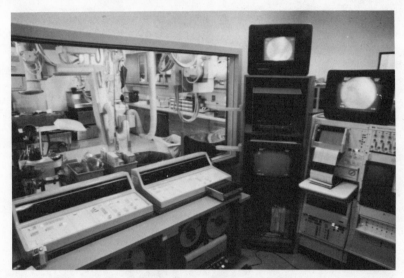

Fig. 2-6.   View of the Interventional Lab Control Room.

specialized ICC technicians for each case 24 hours a day, 7 days a week. Full anesthesia and surgery backup was available at all times.

Patient Selection

Patient selection criteria are as follows: (1) chest pain of <6 hours duration associated with ST segment elevation and (2) ST segment elevation and continued pain of 6–18 hours duration indicating continued myocardial ischemia. Cardiogenic shock, 'cardiopulmonary resuscitation, or potentially reversible coma are not considered contraindications to PTCA. Patients with recent surgery, trauma, or bleeding do not receive thrombolytic therapy but are treated with immediate PTCA alone.

Methods

As soon as the diagnosis of acute myocardial infarction is established, patients receive 1.5 million units of streptokinase dissolved in 250 cc of normal saline administered over 30 minutes. After December of 1985, tissue plasminogen activator (tPA) became available for clinical investigation as part of a combined cooperative protocol between Duke University and University of Michigan. In this study, patients were given tPA instead of streptokinase in a dose of 60 mg during the first hour (10 percent of which was given as an initial bolus) followed by 20 mg in the second hour and 20 mg infused over the third hour.

Each patient was treated with lidocaine, oxygen, Benadryl (50 mg IV), cimetidine (300 mg IV), and IV morphine as needed for pain. Patients were also treated with 1 aspirin and 100 mg of Persantine PO before the procedure and contined on 1 aspirin tid and 25 mg Persantine tid for 6 months after the procedure.

After arrival in the ICC Laboratory, patients are prepped and draped in the usual fashion and an 8 French right femoral venous and arterial sheath are placed in the right groin. A 5 French balloon directed pacing wire is advanced to the inferior vena cava. The pacing wire is advanced to the heart during the case only in the presence of bradydysrhythmias or conduction system disturbances.

The uninvolved coronary artery is studied first to assess the level of collateralization. The infarct related coronary artery is then injected in multiple views. The coronary catheter is then exchanged for a pigtail catheter that is advanced to the ventricle and biplane left ventriculography is performed. An 8 French thinwall PTCA guiding catheter (Interventional Medical) is advanced to the level of the aortic root—a low profile PTCA balloon catheter (Hartzler LPS in 85 percent of cases, Simpson-Robert in 15 percent, ACS). Figure 2-7 shows each component of a standard PTCA system including (1) a guiding catheter, (2) a balloon catheter, (3) a device for administering and regulating pressure within the balloon and (4) a flexible, steerable guidewire. Figure 2-8 shows an example of a patient who had early recanalization of a proximal left anterior descending coronary lesion with a tight residual stenoses after streptokinase (arrow, Panel A). Panel B shows the guidewire and inflated balloon across the obstruction. Following PTCA, the luminal diameter at the site of the previous stenosis appears nearly normal. Although moveable guidewire systems are often used under these circumstances, we have favored the use of a very low profile balloon catheter (Fig. 2-9, Panel A) that is constructed directly onto a guidewire. The system

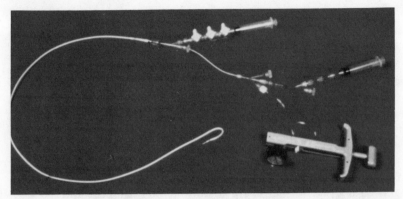

Fig. 2-7. Standard angioplasty equipment including: steerable guide-wire, balloon catheter, guiding catheter, and inflation device. (Courtesy of Advanced Cardiovascular Systems, Inc., Mountain View, CA.

is then steered through the coronary artery from the proximal end of the balloon catheter (Fig. 2-9, Panel B). The rationale for selection of a very low profile catheter is to ease crossing of the obstruction in tight or totally obstructed lesions, and to provide greater visibility of the lesion with diagnostic quality proximal guiding catheter injections.

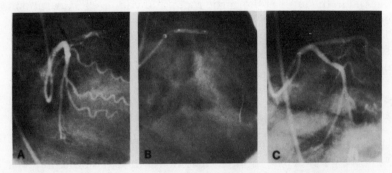

Fig. 2-8. Right anterior oblique projection showing proximal left anterior descending lesion that was successfully recanalized with streptokinase leaving a tight residual stenosis (A, arrow). B shows the balloon during inflation and C shows the final result following PTCA.

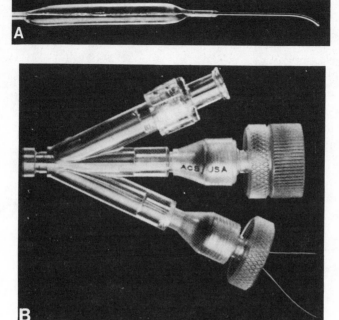

Fig. 2-9. (A) Distal tip of the Hartzlar[R] LPS catheter. (B) Proximal end showing the steering device on the central arm of the manifold. (Courtesy of Advanced Cardiovascular Systems, Inc., Mountain View, CA.

All lesions in the infarct related vessel are dilated during the initial angioplasty. Dilatations are usually performed for a duration of 60 seconds with 6–9 atmospheres applied to each lesion. Results of each dilatation are assessed using proximal guiding catheter injections with high resolution fluoroscopy. Pressure gradients are not recorded. Following the procedure, the patients are returned to the CCU and maintained on heparin overnight.

Occasionally, initially successful dilatations will demonstrate abrupt reclosure during the procedure. Under these circumstances, further dilatations using higher pressures for longer periods of time are applied. If the vessel size permits, larger diameter balloons may be employed if initial repeat dilatations are not successful. Intracoronary nitroglycerin and sublingual

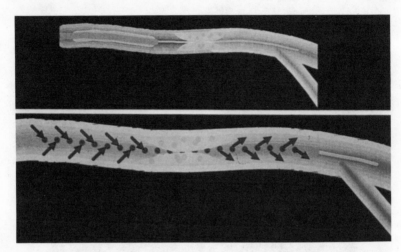

Fig. 2-10. Upper Panel: Illustration of the transluminal reperfusion catheter approaching a totally obstructed lesion after a failed angioplasty. Lower Panel: Blood enters the proximal sideholes, passes through the central lumen, and passes out the distal sideholes to the distal coronary artery.

nifedipine are used to reduce any spastic component to the reocclusion. Intracoronary streptokinase or tPA may be utilized to further dissolve residual coronary thrombus. If all of these measures fail, a "transluminal reperfusion catheter" is inserted (See Fig. 2-10). The preparation and insertion technique for this device is reported elsewhere and will only be briefly reviewed here.[16] The transluminal reperfusion catheter is a catheter-type intracoronary stenting device used to maintain blood flow during transport to emergency surgery after failed angioplasty. Thirty-six sideholes are arranged in a spiral pattern over the distal 10 cm of the catheter. In a failed angioplasty an exchange wire is utilized to remove the original balloon catheter and exchange it for the stenting transluminal reperfusion catheter. This device allows blood to enter the proximal sideholes from the aorta and proximal coronary artery, pass through the area of recurrent occlusion, and pass into the distal coronary, thus allowing immediate relief of ischemia.

Table 2-1
Clinical Characteristics

Total Patients	311
Male/Female	251/60
Age	
Mean (± SD)	57 ± 11 yrs
Range	29–82 yrs
Location of Infarct	
Anterior	137
Inferior	174
Thrombolytic Therapy	
Streptokinase	249
Tissue Plasminogen Activator	40
None	22

Results

From March of 1984 through April of 1986, 311 patients underwent emergency PTCA for acute myocardial infarction (Table 2-1). Two hundred fifty-one patients (81 percent) were male. The mean age was 57 ± 11 years with a range of 29–82 years. The location of the infarct was anterior (including lateral) in 44 percent and inferior (including posterior) in 56 percent. Eighty percent of the patient population received intravenous streptokinase. Thirteen percent of the population received the more recently developed tPA and 7 percent received no thrombolytic therapy due to contraindications such as recent GI bleeding, trauma, or surgery. Results of emergency PTCA are shown in Table 2-2. The wire was able to negotiate the lesion in 99 percent

Table 2-2
Results

% of Lesions crossed with balloon	98%
% of Lesions showing persistent reperfusion after PTCA on final arteriogram	93%
% of Lesions with residual stenosis of ≤ 50%	87%

Table 2-3
Procedural Complications

Death	1%
Stroke	0.6%
Ventricular tachycardia or fibrillation requiring cardioversion	6%
Emergency CABG	5%

of cases. Full balloon placement was achieved in 98 percent. Persistent reperfusion, i.e. full reperfusion of the distal vessels that continued to be present after all dilatations were completed, was present in 93 percent of patients. In some of these patients, however, there was residual thrombus or dissection resulting in a residual luminal narrowing of >50 percent. However, 87 percent of all patients had a residual luminal diameter narrowing of less than or equal to 50 percent following PTCA. The average residual luminal diameter narrowing among all patients with persistent reperfusion following PTCA was 30 ± 6 percent. Procedural complications are shown in Table 2-3. Death occurred in 1.0 percent of patients, stroke in 0.6 percent, cardioversion was required in 6 percent, and emergency CABG in 5 percent.

From the beginning of the helicopter transport system in March of 1985 until April of 1986, 85 patients were transported to the Interventional Lab by helicopter from referring hospitals within 150 miles of Duke University Medical Center. There were 8 episodes of transient hypotension, 4 episodes of V tach, and 4 episodes of severe bradydysrhythmias. Each of these were managed in flight by the Life Flight nurses in continuous radio contact with the Duke cardiologist. Most episodes of hypotension that began in the helicopter were associated with nitroglycerin and/or streptokinase infusion. There were no deaths during transport or during the subsequent angioplasty among this subgroup of patients. The mean air time was 32 ± 13 minutes. This compared to a calculated ground time from point of patient origin to Duke University Medical Center of 131 ± 67 minutes. The average cost to the patient was $518.00 ± $209.00.

Comparison of Streptokinase Alone vs PTCA and Adjunctive Thrombolytic Therapy

A subgroup of 26 consecutive patients with combined emergency PTCA and adjunctive streptokinase therapy were studied with repeat cardiac catheterization prior to discharge using the same protocol as that used during the initial study of regional wall motion in patients receiving streptokinase alone. A composite of the data from each study is shown in Figure 2-11. Patients receiving emergency PTCA again showed a significant improvement in regional wall motion compared to patients who were not reperfused. This improvement was slightly better than in the previous study using streptokinase alone. The overall global ejection fraction was also improved. In the case of patients receiving immediate PTCA, there was just enough additional improvement in the region of the jeopardized myocardium that this became the dominant factor over the reduction in compensa-

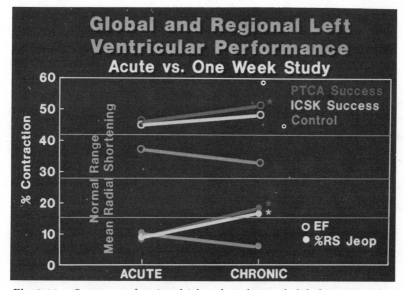

Fig. 2-11. Summary of regional (closed circles) and global (open circles) left ventricular function between the acute and predischarge cardiac catheterization studies.

Table 2-4
Comparison of Streptokinase Alone Versus Thrombolytic
Therapy and PTCA

Outcome	SK	PTCA + Rx
Persistent Reperfusion Rate	62%	93%
% Residual Luminal Narrowing	86%	30%
Mortality Rate (procedural and in-hospital)	17%	11%

tory wall motion. Thus, there now was a statistically significant improvement in global ejection fraction as well as in the regional wall motion among patients receiving immediate PTCA. A summary of the results of the two studies is shown in Table 2-4.

CONCLUSIONS

These data indicate that interventional cardiac catheterization techniques may be applied both safely and effectively on an emergent basis in patients with acute myocardial infarction. Treatment of acute myocardial infarction with thrombolytic agents alone results in a limited initial success rate as well as a significant residual stenosis that is prone to reocclusion. The use of streptokinase therapy results in a reperfusion rate of 30–50 percent while the use of tPA increases the reperfusion rate to 50–70 percent. Despite the limited patency rate, intravenously administered thrombolytic therapy does have the capability of being administered immediately at the referring hospital. Thus a significant number of patients develop reperfusion prior to the angioplasty procedure. Emergency angioplasty allows further reperfusion in a very high percentage of patients (93 percent) coupled with elimination (≤50 percent residual diameter narrowing) in 84 percent.

While emergency PTCA facilities on a 24-hour basis are not practical for many community hospitals, the developement of a dedicated air transport system servicing a wide area around the interventional center assures safe and effective emergency transport of patients at any time of day or night. In patients who are not successfully reperfused following repeated balloon dilatations, the development of the transluminal reperfusion catheter allows continued reperfsuion so that definitive revascularization can be performed safely and effectively using coronary artery bypass grafting. These studies indicate that emergency PTCA may be performed with little or no additional risk in patients with acute myocardial infarction treated with thrombolytic therapy alone. PTCA can now be more widely applied using air transport systems to service local community hospitals. In the minority of patients who do not obtain definitive revascularization with PTCA, the transluminal reperfusion catheter allows persistent reperfusion prior to coronary artery bypass grafting. Finally, immediate PTCA results in a lower residual stenosis than thrombolytic therapy alone (30 percent versus 86 percent) and results in as good or a better improvement in regional and global ventricular peformance compared to thrombolytic therapy alone. The long-term effects of full reperfusion with PTCA on chronic ventricular function and long-term survival are currently being investigated.

REFERENCES

1. Reimer K, Lowe J, Rasmussen M, et al: The wavefront phenomenom of ischemic cell death. I. Myocardial infarct size versus duration of coronary occlusion in dogs. Circulation 56:786–794, 1977
2. Reimer K, Jennings R: The wavefront phenomenon of myocardial ischemic cell death. II. Transmural progression of necrosis within the framework of ischemic bed size (myocardium at risk) and collateral flow. Lab Invest 40:633–644, 1979
3. Theroux P, Ross J, Franklin D, et al: Coronary artery reperfusion. III. Early and late effects on regional myocardial function and dimensions in conscious dogs. Am J Cardiol 38:599–606, 1976
4. Puri PS: Contractile and biochemical effects of coronary reperfusion after extended periods of coronary occlusion. Am J Cardiol 36:244–251, 1975
5. Rentrop P, Blancke H, Karsch R, et al: Selective intracoronary thrombolysis in acute myocardial infarction and unstable angina pectoris. Circulation 63:307–316, 1981
6. Reduto L, Smalling R, Freund G, et al: Intracoronary infusion of streptokinase in patients with acute myocardial infarction. Am J Cardiol 48:403–409, 1981
7. Mathey D, Kuck K, Tilsner V, et al: Nonsurgical coronary artery

recanalization in acute transmural myocardial infarction. Circulation 63:489–497, 1981

8. Stack R, Phillips H, Grierson D, et al: Functional improvement of
    jeopardized myocardium following intracoronary streptokinase in-
    fusion in acute myocardial infarction. J Clin Invest 72:84–95, 1983

9. Kennedy J, Ritchie J, Davis K, et al: Streptokinase in myocardial
    infarction: Western Washington randomized trial of intracoronary
    streptokinase in acute myocardial infarction. New Engl J Med 309:
    1477–1482, 1983

10. Rentrop K, Feit F, Blanke H, et al: Effects of intracoronary strepto-
    kinase and intracoronary nitroglycerin infusion on coronary angi-
    ographic patterns and mortality in patients with acute myocardial
    infarction. New Engl J Med 311:1457–1463, 1984

11. Laffel G, Braunwald E: Thrombolytic therapy: A new strategy for the
    treatment of acute myocardial infarction. New Engl J Med 311:710–
    770, 1984

12. Yusuf S, Collins R, Peto R, et al: Intravenous and intracoronary
    fibrinolytic therapy in acute myocardial infarction: Overview of
    results on mortality, reinfarction and side effects from 33 random-
    ized controlled trials. European Heart Journal 6:556–585, 1985

13. Simoons M, V'D Brand M, DeZwaans C, et al: Improved survival
    after early thrombolysis in acute myocardial infarction. Lancet
    578–581, 1985

14. Gruppo Italiano Per Lo Studio Della Streptochinasi Nell'Infarto
    Miocardico (GISSI). Effectiveness of Intravenous Thrombolytic
    Treatment in Acute Myocardial Infarction. Lancet 397–401, 1986

15. Meyer J, Merx W, Schmitz H, et al: Percutaneous transluminal
    coronary angioplasty immediately after intracoronary streptolysis of
    transmural myocardial infarction. Circulation 66:905, 1982

16. Hinohara T, Simpson J, Phillips H, et al: Transluminal catheter
    reperfusion: A new technique to reestablish blood flow after coro-
    nary occlusion during percutaneous transluminal coronary
    angioplasty. Am J Cardiol 57:683–686, 1986

Reperfusion of the Acute Myocardial Infarction: Role of Anesthesia

Robert A. Kates
Russell Hill
J. G. Reves

Reperfusion of acutely infarcting myocardial tissue is intended to salvage jeopardized myocardium prior to irreversible ischemic injury as well as reduce the morbidity and mortality associated with evolution of the infarction process. Maximal tissue salvage necessitates expedient reperfusion as well as reduction of myocardial metabolic demands prior to reperfusion.

Anesthetic management has a multifaceted impact on patients evolving an acute myocardial infarction. Anesthetic drugs have potent cardiovascular properties that influence myocardial tolerance of ischemia. The anesthesiologist also plays a pivotal role in expediting institution of cardiopulmonary bypass and surgical reperfusion. The role of anesthetic management of patients undergoing nonsurgical myocardial reperfusion in the cardiac catheterization laboratory is also presently being evaluated. In the future, the cardiac anesthesiologist may fill a crucial role

ACUTE REVASCULARIZATION OF THE INFARCTED HEART   ISBN 0-8089-1870-2
Copyright © 1987 by Grune & Stratton, Inc.

during the nonsurgical as well as surgical reperfusion of patients with acute myocardial infarction (AMI).

EFFECT OF ANESTHETIC DRUGS ON THE ISCHEMIC MYOCARDIUM

Inhalation Anesthetics

Historically, the therapeutic effect of anesthetic agents on patients with ischemic heart disease was described 12 years prior to the discovery of the antianginal properties of nitroglycerin. In 1867 Sir Lauder Brunton wrote that "when chloroform was given . . . it relieved the [anginal] pain for the time; but whenever the senses again became clear; the pain was as bad as before."[1]

Within the past 10 years modern anesthetic drugs have been extensively studied to determine their influence on AMI. Anesthetics influence myocardial tolerance of ischemia via direct effects on myocardial tissue and indirectly by changing the hemodynamic correlates of myocardial oxygen supply and demand as well as plasma catecholamine levels (Fig. 3-1).

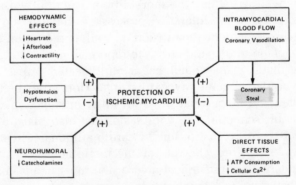

Fig. 3-1. A schematic diagram showing the overall affect of anesthetics during acute myocardial infarction. Note that salvage is achieved by enhancing oxygen delivery and reducing myocardial demand by direct and indrict actions.

CATECHOLAMINES

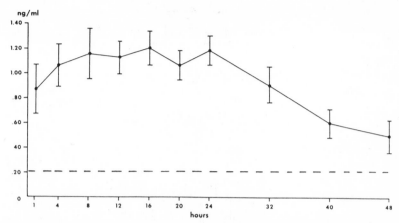

Fig. 3-2. Mean levels ± S.E. of plasma catecholamines in 26 patients related to time of onset of acute chest pain. (Modified from Nadeau RA, deChamplain J: Plasma catecholamines in acute myocardial infarction. Clin Communc. 98:548–554, 1979

Sympathetic overactivity that frequently occurs during acute myocardial infarction (especially anterior infarcts) may accelerate the progression of ischemic injury (Fig. 3-2).[2-4] Detrimental effects of enhanced sympathetic activity on the ischemic heart are usually ascribed to a catecholamine-induced hemodynamic imbalance between oxygen supply and demand. Catecholamines also increase the incidence of serious ventricular arrhythmias, enhance intravascular coagulation, and can increase myocardial fatty acid metabolism that consumes more oxygen than glucose metabolism.[5]

In a chloralose-anesthetized animal study, myocardial catecholamine levels were increased by stimulation of the left stellate ganglion before and after partial coronary artery ligation.[6] Although heart rate did not change and blood pressure increased only slightly, ST-segments were markedly elevated during restricted coronary flow. This demonstrates detrimental effects from catecholamines that are independent of a concommittant increase in external myocardial work, i.e., heart rate and blood pressure. A more recent clinical study demonstrated that the degree of sym-

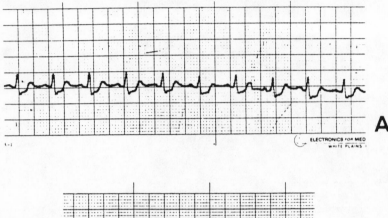

Fig. 3-3. Lead II recordings of a patient with acute coronary artery insufficiency. (A) Before induction of anesthesia, breathing room air. (B) After induction. (Note improvement in ST-segment levels in B tracings.) (Reprinted from Estafanous FG, Viljoen JF: Effect of induction of anesthesia and ventilation on ECG signs of ischemia in patients with acute coronary artery insufficiency. Anesth Analg 53:610–615, 1974. With permission.)

pathoadrenal activity during an acute myocardial infarction correlates with the extent of myocardial damage as well as late mortality.[7]

General anesthesia may prove to be beneficial in acute myocardial infarction patients with high baseline sympathetic tone. This has been shown by the reduction of ST evidence of myocardial ischemia after induction of anesthesia in patients with coronary artery disease (Fig. 3-3). Induction of anesthesia in nonischemic patients with 60 percent nitrous oxide plus enflurane, halothane, or morphine was found to decrease awake

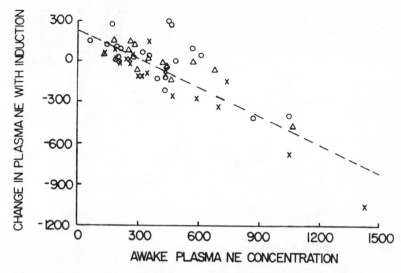

Fig. 3-4. Plasma norepinephrine (NE) concentration (pg/ml) while awake versus changes in plasma NE concentration with induction of anesthesia. Analysis of covariance demonstrated no significant difference among agents; thus, the data for all three agents (x = enflurane, O = halothane, Δ = morphine) were pooled. The line can be described as follows: Change in plasma NE level with induction = (−0.70) (plasma NE level while awake) + 228 (r = 0.83). (Reprinted from Roizen MF, Horrigan RW, Frazer BM: Anesthetic doses blocking adrenergic (stress) and cardiovascular responses to incision-MAC BAR. Anesthesiology 54:390–398, 1981. With permission.)

norepinephrine levels.[8,9] In fact, a positive correlation exists between magnitude of reduction in norepinephrine levels and baseline norepinephrine levels (Fig. 3-4), thus demonstrating that the higher the sympathetic tone the greater the effect of anesthesia induction on catecholamine change.

Increased myocardial work and oxygen consumption due to a hyperdynamic cardiovascular system is detrimental during acute myocardial infarction. Reduction of left ventricular afterload with trimethaphan has been shown to protect jeopardized myocardial tissue in patients with acute myocardial infarction.[10] Enzyme-estimated infarction size, as well as 1-month mortality, was lower in the trimethaphan treated group. Like ganglionic blocking drugs, inhalational anesthetics decrease the hemodynamic corre-

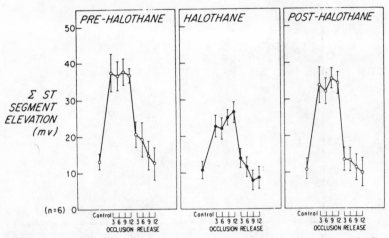

Fig. 3-5. Sum of ST-segment elevations (ΣST) before, during and after 0.75 percent halothane administration in six dogs (Mean $\pm$ SEM). The severity of ischemia produced by occlusion of the identical branch of the left anterior descending coronary artery was significantly (P <.001) less during halothane anesthesia. Reprinted from Bland JHL, Lowenstein E: Halothane-induced decrease in experimental myocardiol ischemia in the non-failing canine heart. Anesthesiology 45:287–293, 1976. With permission.)

lates of myocardial oxygen consumption: heart rate, contractility, and afterload. In a canine coronary artery ligation preparation, the administration of halothane was associated with a decrease in heart rate, systolic arterial pressure, and rate-pressure product (heart rate $\times$ systolic arterial pressure) while left atrial pressure did not change.[11] Summation ST-segment elevation, an index of severity of ischemia, was less during halothane than before or after its administration (Fig. 3-5).[11] In another animal study, halothane administration for 12 hours after coronary ligation significantly reduced myocardial infarction size compared to awake control animals (Fig. 3-6).[12] Coronary ligation in rats resulted in a smaller infarction size during halothane anesthesia compared to fentanyl anesthetized or awake rate.[13] This was partially explained by lower heart rates and blood pressure in the halothane anesthetized group.

Although inhalational anesthetics can beneficially reduce

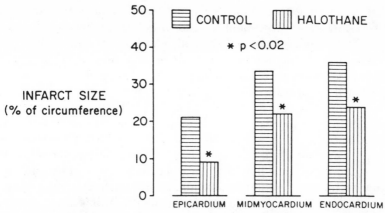

Fig. 3-6. The figure is a comparison of infarct size in halothane-treated and control dogs. Data are expressed as a percentage of the circumference occupied by infarction in the epicardium, mid-myocardium, and endocardium. Asterisk indicates $P < 0.05$ when compared with corresponding control value. Numerical values are 21.6 ± 3.5 versus 8.9 ± 1.9 percent for epicardium, $33.4 \pm$ versus 21.7 ± 2.7 percent for midmyocardium, and 35.9 ± 4.2 versus 23.1 ± 2.9 percent for the endocardium when control data are compared with halothane data, respectively (mean values $\pm$ 1 SEM). (Reprinted from Davis RF, DeBoer LWV, Rude RE, et al: The effect of halothane anesthesia on myocardial necrosis, hemodynamic performance, and regional myocardial blood flow in dogs following coronary artery occlusion. Anesthesiology 59:402–411, 1983. With permission.)

myocardial oxygen consumption, excessive anesthetic-induced myocardial depression and vasodilation may impair coronary perfusion and oxygen balance. In a canine myocardial ischemia model, halothane reduced blood pressure and left ventricular contractility while left ventricular preload was increased and was associated with severe dysfunction in the ischemic myocardial region.[14,15] Hypotension during halothane anesthesia has also been associated with increased infarction size in rats exposed to halothane for 3 hours compared to an awake group.[16] In a subsequent study, however, halothane-induced myocardial depression was greater in normal tissue than in ischemic myocardium.[17] This was postulated to be due to a partial offset of the direct negative inotropic effect of halothane in ischemic tissues by an improvement in myocardial energy balance.[17]

The inhalation anesthetics also influence intramyocardial blood flow. In acutely ischemic dogs, enflurane reduced blood flow to ischemic myocardium to a smaller degree than to normally perfused myocardium.[18]. This relative improvement in oxygen availability-consumption ratio in ischemic tissue was attributed to a reduction in heart rate. In similar animal studies, halothane administration during acute myocardial infarction increased the oxygen availability-consumption ratio in ischemic tissue while it was decreased in a normally perfused region.[12,19] These studies suggest that in the acutely ischemic nonfailing heart, enflurane or halothane may improve oxygenation in jeopardized myocardial tissue.

The potent coronary arterial dilating properties of isoflurane have raised concerns about vasodilation of coronary vascular beds perfusing nonischemic tissue. This can decrease perfusion of ischemic tissue due to coronary steal of intramyocardial blood flow.[20,21] Isoflurane increased total myocardial blood flow in the dog despite a decreased blood pressure and cardiac output.[20] This is in contrast to halothane, which produces similar hemodynamic effects accompanied by a decrease in myocardial blood flow. Presumably, coronary autoregulation was maintained during halothane while the potent vasodilation from isoflurane decoupled myocardial oxygen supply from oxygen consumption (Fig. 3-7). This distinct coronary vascular effect of isoflurane is controversial, however, and other, more recent animal studies demonstrate no evidence of coronary steal physiology from isoflurane.[22,23] In a recent clinical study[24] Tarnow and coworkers found that the administration of isoflurane 0.5 percent in $N_2O:O_2$ (50:50) significantly increased the heart rate required to induce ST changes. These data suggest that inhalation anesthetics are indeed protective and corroborate our earlier observation that higher HR and BP are better tolerated in anesthetized patients than in awake patients during exercise.[25]

Inhalation anesthetics can also directly affect ischemic myocardial tissue. A canine coronary ligation model compared halothane to a similar change in heart rate, blood pressure, and contractility produced with the combination of propranolol and nitroprusside. Despite similar hemodynamics, halothane pro-

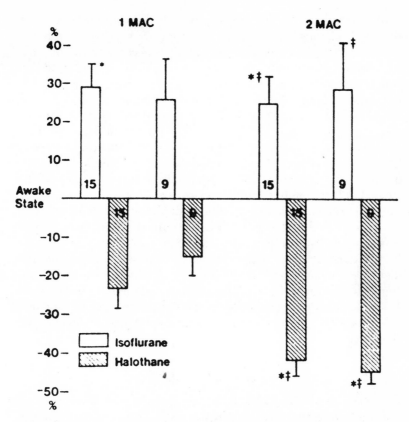

Fig. 3-7. Percent changes in myocardial blood flow determined with 15- and 9-μm spheres during halothane and isoflurane anesthesia (mean ± SEM). *P < 0.05 versus control in corresponding anesthetic; +P < 0.05 versus 1 MAC in corresponding anesthetic; P < 0.05 isoflurane vs halothane in corresponding stages. (Reprinted from Gelman S, Fowler KC, Smith LR: Regional blood flow during isoflurane and halothane anesthesia. Anesth Analg 63:557–565, 1984. With permission.)

duced a greater reduction in severity of myocardial ischemia as determined by summation ST-segment elevation suggesting an additive direct myocardial effect from halothane.[26] We recently evaluated the protective effects of halothane versus pentobarbital (a relatively nondepressant anesthetic) on myocardial tolerance to global ischemia. One hour after halothane 2 percent or

pentobarbital 30 mg/kg^{-1} anesthetic, 12 dogs underwent rapid
cardiac excisions. Left ventricular freewall slabs were prepared
for measurement of time to onset of ischemia contracture (onset of
irreversible ischemic injury) and serial sampling of tissue adeno-
sine triphosphate (ATP) and lactate during normothermic global
ischemia. Ischemic contracture, which is associated with irreversible ischemic injury,[27] was measured as tissue pressure in the
subendocardium and subepicardium with needle-tipped Millar
catheters. Time to onset of contracture was significantly longer in
the halothane than the pentobarbital group for the subendocardium (44.1 ± 1.1 versus 58.1 ± 3.9 minutes, $p < 0.05$) and the
subepicardium (55.6 ± 1.4 versus 68.5 ± 3.1 minutes, $p < 0.05$).
This was accompanied by a reduced depletion rate of tissue ATP
levels in the halothane group (Fig. 3-8). In addition, tissue lactate
was produced at a slower rate in the halothane group. A decrease
in ATP deletion despite no evidence of increased ATP production
(decreased lactate production) suggests a reduction in ATP consumption during ischemia. Since severe ATP depletion (less than
1 n mole/gm wet weight) is associated with irreversible ischemic
tissue damage, halothane may prolong tolerance of myocardial
ischemia.

Intravenous Anesthetics

The intravenous anesthetic drugs have not been as well
investigated as the inhalation drugs with regard to effects on the
ischemic heart. There are, however, a number of studies in man as
well as animals that report effects of intravenous drugs on myocardial oxygen consumption and coronary blood flow in normal
and diseased coronary arteries. The drugs studied are diaze-
pam,[28–31] thiopental,[32,33] ketamine,[34] etomidate,[32,34–36] fentanyl,[37]
and midazolam.[38] A summary of representative human studies is
shown in Figure 3-9. Note that both thiopental and ketamine
increase oxygen consumption (MVO$_2$) as well as coronary blood
flow. The primary reason for the increased MVO$_2$ after thiopental
is an increase in heart rate. The increase in MVO$_2$ is met by an
increase in coronary blood flow (CBF). Likewise, ketamine increases both MVO$_2$ and CBF by increasing heart rate, contractility,
and presumably wall tension. Neither of these drugs is particularly suitable for induction of anesthesia in patients with myocar-

TISSUE ATP LEVELS

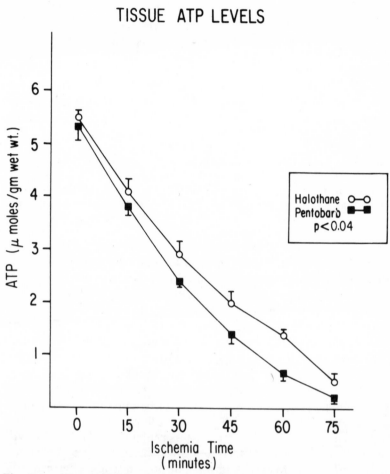

Fig. 3-8. Tissue ATP levels as a function of ischemic time. The rate of ATP degredation was decreased in halothane anesthetized dogs.

dial ischemia because the increases in MVO$_2$ might not be adequately met by CBF in patients with severely compromized coronary artery disease. On the other hand, fentanyl, diazepam, and midazolam all tend to reduce both oxygen consumption and coronary blood flow. Diazepam (.1 mg/kg) has been likened to nitroglycerin in its action on the cardiovascular and coronary

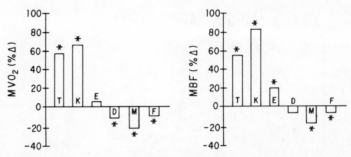

Fig. 3-9. The composite changes in global myocardial oxygen consumption (MVO$_2$) and myocardial blood flow (MBF) measured after thiopental (T), ketamine (K), diazepam (D), midazolam (M), etomidate (E) and fentanyl (F). * = P <.05 value different to predrug control. (Data from Sonntag,[33] Kettler,[34,35] Sonntag,[37] Marty.[38])

artery systems.[29] It appears that midazolam (.2 mg/kg) is similar to diazepam in this regard.[38] Fentanyl (100 mcg/kg) has little effect on coronary hemodynamics although lactate production occurred after fentanyl in five of nine patients with severe coronary artery disease.[37] The most stable coronary and systemic hemodynamics follow etomidate (.3 mg/kg plus infusion of .12 mg/kg/minute). There are virtually no changes in contractility, heart rate, oxygen consumption, or coronary blood flow.[35] On the basis of these studies, etomidate and the two benzodiazepines, midazolam and diazepam, appear to be the superior intravenous anesthetic induction agents. These drugs are, however, devoid of analgesic properties, and stimuli such as tracheal intubation and surgery will undoubtedly increase HR, contractility, and blood pressure, inevitably increasing MVO$_2$. A rational approach to anesthesia would be use of these drugs for induction followed by opiods or inhalation anesthetics during the maintenance of anesthesia.

There are very few studies examining the effects of intravenous agents on experiemental or clinical myocardial ischemia. Thiopental and diazepam were used for the induction of patients with ischemia[39,40] and infarction[40] respectively, but along with methoxyflurane. ST evidence of ischemia disappeared in 16 of 32 (50 percent) patients induced in this manner and ST-segments were reduced 50 percent in 12 of the remaining 16 patients. Presumably the induction of general anesthesia in these patients with acute ischemia lessened ischemia as a result of decreased oxygen demand.[39] Our experience with etomidate in patients having myocardial infarction is that catecholamines are decreased[41] with a consequent reduction in heart rate and blood pressure.

Fentanyl, a potent synthetic opiod, is used commonly for anesthesia in patients with coronary artery disease. The role of fentanyl as a myocardial protective agent has been examined in two laboratory studies. In canine experiments of acute coronary ligation under pentobarbitol and nitrous oxide anesthesia, the administration of fentanyl 25 μg/kg inhibited the release of lactate and inorganic phosphate compared to a prior control ischemic episode.[42] Importantly, this salutory effect was diminished if the heart rate was kept constant during fentanyl. This laboratory study, then, indicates that fentanyl protects the ischemic heart better than no additional anesthesia by slowing the heart rate. In a later study, however, using swine with a 60 percent reduction of coronary blood flow, fentanyl and halothane treated animals had similar degrees of ischemia despite significantly reduced MVO_2 in the halothane treated animals. There were no control swine to show benefit of either of these anesthetic regimens to untreated animals.

Regional Anesthesia

Both spinal and epidural anesthesia have been reported to reduce the amount of myocardial ischemia in man[40] and animals.[43] With both techniques it appears that the underlying mechanism is a reduction of the primary determinants of myocardial oxygen consumption (heart rate, wall tension, and contractility). The efficacy of thoracic epidural anesthesia was demonstrated in a canine model. Epidural anesthesia was associated with reduced ST evidence of ischemia associated with left anterior descending coronary artery (LAD) occlusion and there was also a 46 percent less area of infarction compared to saline control.[43] The primary hemodynamic effect of thoracic epidural anesthesia was a significant ($p < .05$) reduction in HR (18 percent). Thus there was evidence for reduction of myocardial oxygen consumption, but coronary blood flow to the ischemic region was also enhanced ($p < .05$). Whether sympathetic denervation of the heart explains this increased flow is not known. A spinal anesthetic with a sensory level of T7 was recently shown to reduce ST evidence of ischemia in a 73-year-old diabetic man with coronary artery disease.[40] This determinants of myocardial oxygen consumption were reduced presumably because of preganglionic sympathetic denervation. It has been shown that both epidural and spinal anesthesia reduce circulating levels of catecholamines supporting the thesis that reduction in ischemia is mediated by the activity of the sympathetic nervous system.

ANESTHETIC MANAGEMENT OF ACUTE MYOCARDIAL INFARCTION PATIENTS UNDERGOING EMERGENCY SURGICAL REPERFUSION

Emergency coronary artery bypass grafting (CABG) is advocated as a treatment of AMI. The incidence of mortality for emergency CABG in patients with AMI has been reported to be 1–6 percent in several large surgical series.[44–51] There is some evidence that myocardial function may be salvaged by CABG particularly when performed within 4–6 hours of symptom onset,[52,53] and that long-term survival may be improved in some patients.[46,47,54] Likewise there are several reports suggesting that early reperfusion by thrombolysis[55–60] or PTCA[61,62] is potentially valuable in salvaging ischemic myocardium. A significant portion (approximately 6 percent) of thrombolytic or PTCA reperfusion attempts will fail and require emergency CABG. Large prospective randomized trials have not been reported to firmly establish the proper role of each option in conjunction with conventional medical therapy.[63,64] The merits of each of these treatment modalities is discussed elsewhere in this monograph. It is predictable, however, that early aggressive interventions will increase in frequency and therefore place anesthesiologists in a prominant role of caring for patients with AMI undergoing emergency CABG as both a primary therapy and following unsuccessful reperfusion with PTCA or thrombolysis.

The anesthetic management of these patients involves several considerations not normally associated with elective CABG patients. These include the rapid assessment and transport of sometimes hemodynamically unstable patients to a hastily prepared operating room, management of the full stomach in nonfasting patients, establishment of adequate monitoring in patients who have been anticoagulated, and postoperative care of patients with AMI. The treatment of acute myocardial ischemia, cardiac failure, serious ventricular dysrhythmias, and bleeding complications is potentially more demanding in AMI patients than elective CABG patients. To attempt to more precisely define management problems or risks in this patient group, we conducted a retrospective study comparing the perioperative courses of patients undergoing emergency CABG during AMI with patients undergoing elective CABG. The results have been published elsewhere,[65] but will be reviewed here.

Comparison of AMI and Elective Patients Undergoing CABG

Twenty-three patients who underwent emergency CABG during AMI over an 18-month period were identified from a computer generated data bank of all cardiac surgical patients at Duke University Medical Center. Criteria for inclusion in the study were documentation of the onset of persistant chest pain within 12 hours of induction of anesthesia and associated ST-segment elevation of at least 0.2 mV on 2 or more leads of a standard 12-lead ECG. Using the same computerized data bank the AMI patients were individually matched for gender, operating surgeon, similar preoperative angiographic ejection fraction (within an average of 8 percent), and aortic cross clamp time (within an average of 12 minutes) with 23 patients who underwent elective CABG over the same time period.

AMI patients were transported to the earliest available operating room following catheterization. Intravenous access, ECG, and direct arterial blood pressure monitoring were quickly established. Pulmonary artery catheterization via an internal or external jugular vein was performed in all AMI patients either before or after induction of anesthesia depending on readiness of the surgical staff. In elective patients all monitoring devices were placed prior to induction of anesthesia. The anesthetic agents chosen and vasoactive and antiarrhythmic drugs were used at the discretion of the individual anesthesiologist. The anesthesiologists were the same in both groups. All patients underwent coronary revascularization during a single period of elective cardiac arrest using cold potassium cardioplegia with the aorta clamped. Each surgeon followed his customary operative management in both groups. Following surgery, patients were taken to the cardiac surgical intensive care unit for postoperative mechanical ventilation and hemodynamic monitoring.

Preoperative patient characteristics, anesthetic agents, antianginal, inotropic, and antiarrhythmic drug usage, cardiac index, activated clotting times, blood administration, postoperative bleeding, and perioperative complications were compared between groups. The 23 AMI patients were anesthetized 6 ± 3.0 (range 1.5–11.0) hours after the onset of chest pain. Fifteen AMI patients had emergency streptokinase therapy and, in addition to streptokinase, seven had attempted PTCA prior to CABG. In the immediate preoperative period, the AMI patients required treatment for cardiac failure and hypotension with inotropes (4 versus 0; p < .05) and use of intraaortic baloon counter pulsation (IABP) (9 versus 0; p < .005) more often. They also needed acute antianginal therapy with intravenous nitroglycerin (22 versus 1; p < .005) and IABP, and treatment of ventricular dysrhythmias with intravenous lidocaine (13 versus 1; p < .005) more frequently.

In nonfasting AMI patients, anesthesia was induced with etomidate, fentanyl, and succinylcholine followed by immediate intubation. Otherwise, anesthetic agents for the two groups were similar. A narcotic (fentanyl or sufentanil), muscle relaxant (pancuronium or vecuronium) and inhalation (halothane or enflurane) combination was predominantly used.

Inotropic and antiarrhythmic drugs were used more frequently in the AMI group both before and after cardiopulmonary bypass (Table 3-1). The length of aortic clamp time and total cardiopulmonary bypass time was similar for both groups. The number of coronary ateries grafted and the cardiac index at the end of surgery were also similar. There were no intraoperative deaths.

Three (13 percent) AMI patients died postoperatively. Two patients died of cardiac arrest following prolonged cardiac output on the first and second postoperative days. The third died on postoperative day 49 with respiratory failure and sepsis. There

Table 3-1
Intraoperative Data

	AMI	(N)	Elective	(N)	P
Antiarrhythmics* Before Bypass	14	(23)	1	(23)	<.005
Antiarrhythmics* After Bypass	16	(23)	5	(23)	<.005
Inotropes[†] Before Bypass	3	(23)	0	(23)	<.10
Inotropes[†] After Bypass	12	(23)	3	(23)	<.005
Nitroglycerin Before Bypass	23	(23)	22	(23)	NS
Nitroglycerin After Bypass	16	(23)	17	(23)	NS
Nitroprusside Before Bypass	5	(23)	8	(23)	NS
Nitroprusside After Bypass	15	(23)	17	(23)	NS
IABP	9	(23)	0	(23)	<.005
Aortic Clamp Time (min)	38.9 ± 23	(23)	43.0 ± 16	(23)	NS
Bypass Time (min)	103 ± 46	(23)	103 ± 29	(23)	NS
Number of Grafts	2.91 ± 1.6	(23)	2.65 ± .93	(23)	NS
Cardiac Index at end of Procedure ($1/min/m^2$)	2.48 ± .64	(23)	2.53 ± .45	(23)	NS

* lidocaine, procainamide, or bretylium
† dopamine, epinephrine, or norepinephrine

was no hospital mortality in the elective group. Electrocardiograms one day after surgery revealed new Q waves in 15 and sustained ST-segment elevation in 3 AMI patients. Three AMI patients without postoperative ECG evidence of a myocardial infarction had significant elevation of CK-MB isoenzymes. Two AMI patients had no postoperative electrocardiograms or CK-MB isoenzymes levels available for review. Only one elective patient had new Q waves on a postoperative ECG. The AMI group required postoperative inotropic support more often and tended to have a higher incidence of serious dysrhythmias than did the elective group (Table 3-2). The number of patients requiring prolonged postoperative ventilation (>24 hours) and extended ICU care (>2 days) was significantly higher in the AMI group (Table 3-2).

Of particular interest was the postoperative blood loss from chest tube drainage in the first 12 hours, which was greater in patients given streptokinase therapy (1290 ± 610 versus 842 ±

Table 3-2
Postoperative Variables

	AMI	(N)	Elective	(N)	P
Intravenous Drugs					
Inotropes	15	(23)	4	(23)	<.005
Vasodilators	23	(23)	23	(23)	NS
Antiarrhythmics	18	(23)	9	(23)	<.01
Dysrhythmias					
Atrial Fibrillation	9	(23)	5	(23)	NS
Ventricular Tachycardia	1	(23)	0	(23)	NS
Ventricular Fibrillation	3	(23)	0	(23)	<.10
3· AV Block	1	(23)	0	(23)	NS
Intubated > 24 hours	10	(23)	1	(23)	<.005
ICU Stay > 2 days	9	(23)	3	(23)	<.05
Death	3	(23)	0	(23)	<.10
Reexploration	1	(23)	2	(23)	NS
Neurological Deficit	2	(23)	0	(23)	NS
Prolonged Low C.O.	3	(23)	1	(23)	NS
Mediastinitis	2	(23)	0	(23)	NS

470 cc; p=.03) compred to their matched cohorts. Activated clotting times, measured intraoperatively before heparin administration (159 ± 98 versus 126 ± 110 ± 21 sec; p = .09) and after heparin reversal with protamine (171 ± 98 versus 126 ± 37 sec; p = .10) tended to be greater in those patients who had streptokinase. Blood utilization also tended to be higher in these patients (8.7 ± 5.0 versus 6.3 ± 2.5 units; p = .10). Five streptokinase patients received aminocaproic acid intraoperatively without altering blood usage (8.0 ± 4.1 versus 9.1 ± 5.6 units) or chest tube drainage (1237 ± 727 versus 1314 ± 589cc) compared to the 10 who did not.

   Thus in these patients that had the same operation by the same surgeons and similar anesthetic treatment by the same anesthesiologists, there are significantly increased risks associated with AMI. Patients with AMI came to the operating room with inotropic and IABP support more often than the elective patients. Importantly, induction of general anesthesia did not increase this need. The interval from induction to cardiopulmonary bypass was free of new inotropic interventions in the AMI group. There was, however, a much more frequent requirement for inotropic support necessary for discontinuation of cardiopulmonary bypass in the AMI group. This suggests that myocardial ischemia prior to bypass leads to poor tolerance of hypothermic cardiac arrest with cardioplegia. The postoperative course for the AMI group is more complex as indicated by increased frequency of prolonged ventilation and ICU care, although the incidence of individual complications was not statistically different from the elective group.

Thrombolytic therapy prolongs the ACT and leads to more postoperative hemorrhage and blood requirements. Phillips et al[51] also found a greater difference in blood usage between patients who had streptokinase therapy immediately before surgery and elective patients (8.5 versus 1.5 units). Streptokinase indirectly activates the endogenous fibrinolytic system by combining with the proactivator of plasminogen to form an activator complex that then catalyzes the conversion of circulating plasminogen into plasmin. Plasmin is capable of lysing fresh clots and digesting clotting factors V, VIII, prothrombin, and fibrinogen. Streptokinase produces an excess of plasmin, resulting in a systemic lytic state.[66] Aminocaproic acid is the recommended antidote for complications of streptokinase therapy. In our experience, however, there were no differences in bleeding between 5 of our thrombolytic patients who received aminocaproic acid intraoperatively and the remaining 10 who did not. The role of aminocaproic acid in the reversal of streptokinase needs further study.

Since patients with AMI represent greater anesthetic and surgical risk, anesthesiologists caring for these patients during CABG are in a position to help minimize myocardial damage prior to surgical revascularization. Patient transfer from the cardiologist's care to the operating room should be expedited as quickly and smoothly as is possible to minimize ischemic time. Pharmacologic manipulations should be optimized to increase collateral coronary perfusion and minimize myocardial metabolic demands. Intra-aortic baloon counterpulsation may be of benefit in cases of hemodynamic instability or unavoidable delays in operating room availability.[67] Routine prophylatic antiarrhythmic therapy is recommended. Extensive hemodynamic monitoring is valuable in these potentially unstable patients but every effort should be made not to delay the start of surgery. Extra caution by experienced personnel is required for central cannulation in anticoagulated patients to prevent bleeding and hematoma formation at catheterization sites.

ANESTHESIA MANAGEMENT FOR
NONSURGICAL MYOCARDIAL REPERFUSION

Nonsurgical myocardial revascularization with percutaneous transluminal coronary angioplasty (PTCA) and streptokinase is being used to restore myocardial perfusion during acute myocardial infarction.[68,69] Optimal patient management during this procedure presents a clinical challenge. Pain, anxiety, and reflex-increased sympathetic tone resulting in tachycardia and hypertension frequently occurs and can accelerate the progression of ischemic myocardial injury. Furthermore, increased parasympathetic tone can produce heart block and emesis. The development of hemodynamic instability in these nonfasting patients increases the risk of pulmonary aspiration of gastric contents. Since general anesthesia can reduce plasma catecholamine and tracheal intubation can decrease the risk of pulmonary aspiration and improve ventilation, we recently evaluated the effects of general anesthesia during emergency PCTA for acute myocardial infarction.[70]

Criteria for entry into the emergency PTCA protocol included onset of ischemic pain within 6 hours and ST-segment elevation sof 2 mm or greater. Patients received streptokinase 1.5 million units IV, lidocaine 225 mg IV in divided injections followed by a 2.0 mg · min^{-1}, and heparin 10,000 units IV. They underwent urinary bladder catheterization and percutaneous cannulation of the right femoral artery and vein. Following placement of a transvenous pacing catheter, diagnostic left ventriculography, and coronary arteriography, the occluding lesion was dilated.

After informed, written consent, six consecutive patients received general anesthesia for the emergency PCTA proceedure. Direct arterial blood pressure and ECG were monitored and one arterial blood sample was drawn beween venticulography and angioplasty. Fentanyl 100–150 μg IV and pancuronium 1.0 mg IV preceeded induction with etomidate 0.3 mg · kg^{-1} IV and succinylcholine 1.5 mg · kg^{-1} IV. Rapid-sequence endotracheal intubation was followed by cannulation of the right groin and the

PTCA procedure. Ventilation was controlled. Anesthesia was maintained with enflurane 0.3 percent, nitrous oxide 50 percent, and vecuronium 0.05 mg · kg^{-1} IV. Upon termination of the procedure, the anesthetic was discontinued and with the return of consciousness, the trachea was extubated. After these six patients, standard patient management was reinstituted, which consisted of nasal cannula oxygen (5 1 · min^{-1}) and morphine 0–10 mg IV plus local infiltration with lidocaine 1 percent in the right groin. An anesthesiologist observed and recorded hemodynamic measurements during the next six consecutive patients. All patients were interviewed after the procedure to evaluate patient assessment of the program.

During general anesthesia the heart rate and rate-pressure product were significantly below baseline levels and remained reduced throughout the procedure while hemodynamic values in the awake group did not change (Fig. 3-10). Arterial oxygen tension was higher in the anesthesized group (238 ± 91 versus 65 ± 17 mmHg, p < 0.002) while $PaCO_2$ (40.8 ± 6.6, 37.0 ± 4.1 mmHg) and pH (7.36 ± 0.02, 7.35 ± 0.05) were similar between groups. No anesthetic related complications were encountered. Patient assessments demonstrated that all awake patients were in moderate discomfort whereas none of the anesthetized patients recalled any procedural events.

This initial experience indicates that general anesthesia can be safely administered to patients undergoing emergency PTCA during acute myocardial infarction. The potential advantages of this anesthetic technique is the reduction in heart rate-blood pressure product and improvement in arterial oxygenation that may favorably affect myocardial oxygen supply/ demand balance. Although previous reports have evaluated the beneficial effects of parenteral analgesia[71] and sedation,[72] including inhalation of nitrous oxide,[73] general anesthesia during acute myocardial infarction in nonsurgical patients has not been previously evaluted.

No serious anesthetic complications developed in these six cases; however, general anesthesia for emergency PTCA during acute myocardial infarction is not without potential risks. Increased anesthetic risks may be due to the emergent nature of the procedure, the patient's cardiac disease, and preinduction streptokinase therapy. Presently, our contraindications for general

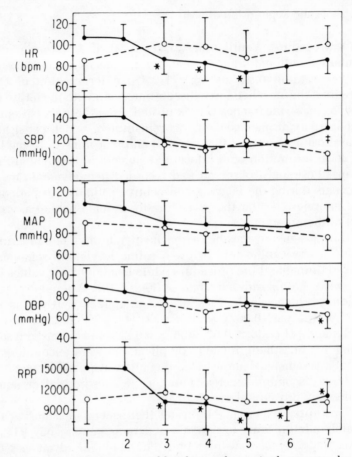

Fig. 3-10. Hemodynamic variables during the angioplasty procedure in the anesthetized (filled circles, solid line) and in the awake group (open circles, dashed line). Measurements are (1) baseline, i.e., upon arrival in the laboratory and before anesthetic induction; (2) 5 minutes after tracheal intubation; (3) immediately prior to ventriculography; (4) after ventriculography; (5) at myocardial reperfusion; (6) at extubation; (7) 5 minutes after extubation, or final measurement in awake group. Abbreviations: HR, heart rate; SBP, systolic arterial blood pressure; MAP, mean arterial blood pressure; DBP, diastolic arterial blood pressure; RPP, rate-pressure product (HR × SBP). *P < 0.05 from baseline, ‡P < 0.05 between groups. Reprinted from Kates RA, Stack RS, Hill RF, et al: General anesthesia for patients undergoing percutaneous transluminal coronary angioplasty during acute myocardial infarction. Anes Analg 65:815–818, 1986. With permission.

anesthesia during emergency PTCA for acute myocardial infarction are the anticipation of difficulty with oral endotracheal intubation and noncardiac disease that would substantially increase anesthetic risk. Bradyrhythmias and hypotension should be treated prior to anesthetic induction; however, patients with severe hemodynamic instability might require tracheal intubation to prevent aspiration and to normalize ventilation. Hyperoxic mechanical ventilation, which signficantly improved oxygenation in our patients, may benefit ischemic myocardial border zones. A considerable number of patients with acute myocardial infarction have been shown to be hypoxemic,[74] which can extend ischemic injury and infarction size. Increased oxygen availability to ischemic border zones decreases ischemic in dogs receiving hyperoxic mixtures.[75,76] Finally, since time from coronary artery occlusion to reperfusion is of utmost importance, anesthesia must not prolong, but facilitate the procedure.

Although definitive conclusions cannot be drawn from this initial experience, we are encouraged by the decrease in heart rate-blood pressure product in the anesthetized group and the fact that anesthesia administration did not increase the time required for reperfusion. The complete relief of pain and enhancement of oxygenation are all advantages of this technique. Randomized clinical studies are now in order to definitively test the hypothesis that general anesthesia can augment nonsurgical and pharmacologic salvage of ischemic myocardium during acute myocardial infarction.

CONCLUSION

The anesthesiologist clearly performs a multifaceted role in the management of patients with acute myocardial infarction. Experimental evidence indicates potential advantageous cardiovascular effects of anesthetic drugs that can theoretically improve myocardial salvage. Management of the emergency patient with acute myocardial infarction can maintain hemodynamic stabilization and facilitate surgical reperfusion. In the future, the anesthesiologist may also participate in nonsurgical reperfusion procedures to optimize patients management and improve myocardial salvage.

REFERENCES

1. Brunton TL: Use of Nitrite of Amyl in Angina Pectoris. Lancet 2: 97–98, 1867
2. Waldenstrom AP, Hjalmarson AC, Thornell L: A possible role of noradrenaline in the development of myocardial infarction. Am Heart J 95:(1)43–51, 1978
3. Nadeau RA, deChamplain J: Plasma catecholamines in acute myocardial infarction. Clin Communic 98:548–554, 1979
4. Daniell HB, Webb JG, Privitera PJ: Studies of the interrelationship between plasma norepinephrine, plasma renin activity and acute myocardial infarction in dogs. Res Comm Chem Path Pharm 20:289–302, 1978
5. Opie LH: Mebabolism of free fatty acids, glucose and catecholamines in acute myocardial infarction. Am J Cardio 36:938–953, 1975
6. Raab W, Van Lith P, Lepeschkin E, et al: Catecholamine-induced myocardial Hypoxia in the presence of impaired coronary dilatability independent of external cardiac work. Am J Cardiol 9:455–470, 1962
7. Karlsberg R, Cryer PE, Roberts R: Serial plasma catecholamine response early in the course of clinical acute myocardial infarction: Relationship to infarct extent and mortality. Am Heart J 102:(1)24–29, 1981
8. Kono K, Philbin DM, Coggins CH, et al: Renal function and stress response during halothane or fentanyl anesthesia. Anesth Analg 60:(8)552–556, 1981
9. Roizen MF, Horrigan RW, Frazer BM: Anesthetic doses blocking adrenergic (stress) and cardiovascular responses to incision-MAC BAR. Anesthesiology 54:390–398, 1981
10. Shell WE, Sobel BE: Protection of jeopardized ischemic myocardium by reduction of ventricular afterload. New Engl J Med 291:(10)481–486, 1974
11. Bland JHL, Lowenstein E: Halothane-induced decrease in experimental myocardial ischemia in the non-failing canine heart. Anesthesiology 45:287–293, 1976
12. Davis RF, DeBoer LWV, Rude RE, et al: The effect of halothane anesthesia on myocardial necrosis, hemodynamic performance, and regional myocardial blood flow in dogs following coronary artery occlusion. Anesthesiology 59:402–411, 1983
13. MacLeod BA, Augereau P, Walker MJA: Effects of halothane anesthesia compared with fentanyl anesthesia and no anesthesia during coronary ligation in rats. Anesthesiology 58:44–52, 1983

14. Lowenstein E, Foex P, Francis CM, et al: Regional ischemic ventricular dysfunction in myocardium supplied by a narrowed coronary artery with increasing halothane concentration in the dog. Anesthesiology 55:349–359, 1981

15. Francis CM, Foex P, Lowenstein E, et al: Interaction between regional myocardial ischaemia and left ventricular performance under halothane anaesthesia. Br J Anaesth 54:965–979, 1982

16. Kissin I, Stanbridge R, Bishop SP, et al: Effect of halothane on myocardial infarct size in rats. Canad Anaesth Soc J 28:(3)239–243, 1981

17. Kissin I, Thomson CT, Smith LR: Effect of halothane on contractile function of ischemic myocardium. J Cardiovasc Pharm 4:438–442, 1983

18. Smith G, Evans DH, Asher MJ, et al: Enflurane improves the oxygen supply/demand balance in the acutely ischaemic canine myocardium. Acta Anaesthesiol Scand 24:44–47, 1982

19. Smith G, Rogers K, Thorburn J: Halothane improves the balance of oxygen supply to demand in acute experimental myocardial ischaemia. Br J Anaesth 52:577–583, 1980

20. Gelman S, Fowler KC, Smith LR: Regional blood flow during isoflurane and halothane anesthesia. Anesth Analg 63:557–565, 1984

21. Merin RG, Lowenstein E, Gelman S: Is anesthesia beneficial for the ischemic heart? III. Anesthesiology 64:(2)137–140, 1986

22. Cason BA, Verrier E, London MJ, et al: Effects of isoflurane and halothane on coronary vascular resistance and collateral blood flow. Anesthesiology 63:(3A)A16, 1985

23. Gilbert M, Roberts SL, Blomberg RW, et al: Greater coronary reserve in swine anesthetized with isoflurane vs halothane. Anesthesiology 63:(3A)A15, 1985

24. Tarnow J, Markschies-Hornung A, Schulte-Sasse U: Isoflurane improves the tolerance to pacing-induced myocardial ischemia. Anesthesiology 64:147–156, 1986

25. Reves JG, Samuelson PN, Lell WA, et al: Violation of RPP exercise threshold in coronary patients. Anesthesiology 51:S64, 1979.

26. Gerson JI, Hickey RF, Bainton CR: Treatment of myocardial ischemia with halothane or nitroprusside-propranolol. Anesth Analg 61:10–14, 1982

27. Lowe JE, Cummings RG, Adams DH, et al: Evidence that ischemic cell death begins in the subendocardium independent of variations in collateral flow or wall tension. Circulation 68:190, 1983

28. Formanek A, Korbuly D, Moore R, et al: The effect of valium on myocardial blood flow. Diag Radiology 121:541–544, 1976

29. Daniell HB: Cardiovascular effects of diazepam and chlordiazepoxide. Eur J Pharm 32:58–65, 1975

30. Cote P, Gueret P, Bourassa MG: Systemic and coronary hemodynamic effects of diazepam in patients with normal and diseased coronary arteries. Circulation 50:1210–1216, 1974

31. Ikram H, Rubin AP, Jewkes RF: Effect of diazepam on myocardial blood flow of patients with and without coronary artery disease. Br Heart J 35:626–630, 1973

32. Patschke D, Bruckner JB, Gethmann JW, et al: Comparison of the immediate effects of etomidate, propanidid and thiopentone on haemodynamics, coronary bloodflow and myocardial oxygen consumption: An experimental study. Acta Anaesthesiologica Belgica N2-3:112–119, 1975

33. Sonntag H, Hellberg K, Schenk H-D, et al: Effects of thiopental (Trapanal) on coronary blood flow and myocardial metabolism in man. Acta anaesth scand 19:69–78, 1975

34. Kettler D, Sonntag H, Wolfram-Donath U, et al: Haemodynamics, myocardial function, oxygen requirement, and oxygen supply of the human heart after administration of etomidate, in Doenicke A (ed.): Anaesthesiology and Resuscitation. Berlin, Springer-Verlag, 1977, pp 81–94

35. Kettler D, Sonntag H, Donath U, et al: Hamodynamik, myokardmechanik, sauerstoffbedarf und sauerstoffversorgung des menschlichen herzens unter narkosccinlcitung mit etomidate. Anaesthesist 23:116–121, 1974

36. Prakash O, Dhasmana KM, Verdouw PD, et al: Cardiovascular effects of etomidate with emphasis on regional myocardial blood flow and performance. Br J Anaesth 53:591–599, 1981

37. Sonntag H, Larsen R, Hilfike, et al: Myocardial blood flow and oxygen consumption during high-dose fentanyl anesthesia in patients with coronary artery disease. Anesthesiology 56:417–422, 1982

38. Marty J, Nitenberg A, Blanchet F, et al: Effects of midazolam on the coronary circulation in patients with coronary artery disease. Anesthesiology 64:206–210, 1986

39. Estafanous FG, Viljoen JF: Effect of induction of anesthesia and ventilation on ECG signs of ischemia in patients with acute coronary artery insufficiency. Anesth Analg 53:610–615, 1974

40. Viljoen JF, Estafanous FG, Kim KS: Anaesthesia for emergency coronary artery surgery. Br J Anaesth 46:953–960, 1974

41. McIntyre RW, Kates RA, Clements F, et al: The effect of a general anesthesia on the stress response to acute myocardial infarction. (Abstract) Anesthesiology 65:A48, 1986

42. van der Vusse GJ, van Belle H, van Geven W, et al: Acute effect of fentanyl on haemodynamics and myocardial carbohydrate utilization and phosphate release during ischaemia. Br J Anaesth 51:927–935, 1979

43. Davis RF, DeBoer LWV, Maroko PR: Thoracic epidural anesthesia reduces myocardial infarct size after coronary artery occlusion in dogs. Anesth Analg 65:711–717, 1986

44. Berg R Jr, Selinger SL, Leonard JJ, et al: Acute evolving myocardial infarction: A surgical emergency. J Thorac Cardiovasc Surg 88:902–906, 1984

45. DeWood MA, Spores J, Berg R Jr, et al: Acute myocardial infarction: a decade of experience with surgical reperfusion in 701 patients. Circulation 68:(suppl II) II-8 – II-16, 1983

46. Berg R Jr, Selinger SL, Leonard JJ, et al: Immediate coronary artery bypass for acute evolving myocardial infarction. J Thorac Cardiovasc Surg 81:493–497, 1981

47. Selinger SL, Berg R Jr, Leonard JJ, et al: Surgical treatment of acute evolving anterior myocardial infarction. Circulation 64:(suppl II) II-28 – II-33, 1981

48. Phillips SJ, Kongtahworn C, Zeff RH, et al: Emergency coronary artery revascularization: a possible therapy for acute myocardial infarction. Circulation 60:(2)241–246, 1979

49. DeWood MA, Spores J, Notski RN, et al: Medical and surgical management of myocardial infarction. Am J Cardiol 44:1356–1364, 1979

50. Berg R Jr, Kendall RW, Duvoisin GE, et al: Acute myocardial infarction: a surgical emergency. J Thorac Cardiovasc Surg 70:(3) 432–439, 1975

51. Phillips SJ, Zeff RH, Skinner JR, et al: Reperfusion protocol and results in 738 patients with evolving myocardial infarction. Ann Thorac Surg 41:119–125, 1986

52. VanHaecke J, Flameng W, Sergeant P, et al: Emergency bypass surgery: late effects on size of infarction and ventricular function. Circulation 72:(suppl II)II-179 – II-184, 1985

53. DeWood MA, Heit J, Spores J, et al: Anterior transmural myocardial infarction: effect of surgical coronary reperfusion on global and regional left ventricular function. J Am Coll Cardiol 1:(5)1123–1134, 1983

54. Kirklin JK, Blackstone EH, Zorn GL, et al: Intermediate-term results of coronary artery bypass grafting for acute myocardial infarction. Circulation 72:(suppl II)II-175 – II-178, 1985

55. Laffel GL, Braunwald E: Thrombolytic Therapy: a new strategy for

the treatment of acute myocardial infarction. N Engl J Med 311:(11)710–717, 1984

56. Laffel GL, Braunwald E: Thrombolytic Therapy: a new strategy for the treatment of acute myocardial infarction. (Part Two) N Engl J Med 311:(12)770–776, 1984

57. Stack RS, Phillips HR, Grierson DS, et al: Functional improvement of jeopardized myocardium following intracoronary streptokinase infusion in acute myocardial infarction. J Clin Inves 72:84–95, 1983

58. Kennedy JW, Ritchie JL, Davis KB, et al: Western Washington randomized trial of intracoronary streptokinase in acute myocardial infarction. N Engl J Med 309:(24)1477–1482, 1983

59. Spann JF, Sherry S, Carabello BA, et al: Coronary thrombolysis by intravenous streptokinase in acute myocardial infarction: acute and follow-up studies. Am J Cardiol 53:655–661, 1984

60. Collen D, Topol EJ, Tiefenbrunn AJ, et al: Coronary thrombolysis with recombinant human tissue-type plasminogen activator: a prospective, randomized, placebo-controlled trial. Circulation 70:(6) 1012–1017, 1984

61. Pepine CJ, Prida X, Hill JA, et al: Percutaneous transluminal coronary angioplasty in acute myocardial infarction. Am Heart J 107:820–822, 1984

62. O'Neill W, Timmis GC, Dourdillon PD, et al.; A prospective randomized clinical trial of intracoronary streptokinase versus coronary angioplasty for acute myocardial infarction. N Engl J Med 314:812–818, 1986

63. McIntosh HD, Buccino RA: Emergency coronary artery revascularization of patients with acute myocardial infarction: You can. . .but should you? Circulation 60:(2)247–250, 1979

64. Braunwald E: The aggressive treatment of acute myocardial infarction. Circulation 71:(6)1087–1092, 1985

65. Hill RF, Kates RA, Davis D, et al: Anesthetic implications for the management of patients with acute myocardial infarction: A matched cohort study of patients undergoing emergency CABG Operations (Abstract) Anes Analg (in press)

66. Sharma GVRK, Cella G, Parisi AF, et al: Thrombolytic therapy. N Engl J Med 306:1268–1276, 1982

67. Murphy DA, Craver JM, Jones EL, et al: Surgical management of acute myocardial ischemia following percutaneous transluminal coronary angioplasty. J Thorac Cardiovasc Surg 87:332–339, 1984

68. Holmes J DR, Smith HC, Vlietstra RE, et al: Percutaneous transluminal coronary angioplasty, alone or in combination with streptokinase therapy, during acute myocardial infarction. Mayo Clin Proc 60:449–456, 1985

69. Meyer J, Merx W, Schmitz H, et al: Percutaneous transluminal coronary angioplasty immediately after intracoronary streptolysis of transmural myocardial infarction. Circulation 66:(5)905–915, 1982

70. Kates RA, Stack RS, Hill RF, et al: General anesthesia for patients undergoing percutaneous transluminal coronary angioplasty during acute myocardial infarction. Anes Analg 65:815–818, 1986

71. Grossman JA, Enselberg CD: A clinical trial of pentazocine analgesia in acute myocardial infarction and acute coronary insufficiency. Curr Thera Res 13:505–511, 1971

72. Calvert A, Mitchell AS, Sinclair G: A double-blind evaluation of diazepam and amylobarbitone in acute myocardial infarction. Med J Aust 2:624–627, 1974

73. Thompson PL, Lown B: Nitrous oxide as an analgesic in acute myocardial infarction. JAMA 235:924–927, 1976

74. Valentine PA, Fluck DC, Mounsey JPD, et al: Blood-gas changes after acute myocardial infarction. Lancet 2:837–841, 1966

75. Sayen JJ, Sheldon WF, Horwitz O, et al: Studies of coronary disease in the experimental animal: II. Polarographic determinations of local oxygen availability in the dog's left ventricle during coronary occlusion and pure oxygen breathing. J Clin Invest 30:932–940, 1951

76. Maroko PR, Radvany P, Braunwald E, et al: Reduction of infarct size by oxygen inhalation following acute coronary occlusion. Circulation 52:360–368, 1975

Intervention in Acute Myocardial Infarction: The Role of Surgical Management

Robert A. Guyton, David A. Langford,
Joseph M. Arcidi, Jr., Douglas C. Morris,
Henry A. Liberman, Charles R. Hatcher, Jr.

HISTORICAL PERSPECTIVE

Myocardial infarction has been a particular source of frustration for surgeons. Coronary occlusion is a mechanical problem and surgeons are trained to attack and repair mechanical problems. In the late 1960s and early 1970s surgeons, in typical fashion, made desperate attempts to save desperately ill patients. The intra-aortic balloon pump allowed transportation and catheterization of patients in cardiogenic shock and emergency revascularization was attempted. Salvage, especially in patients with massive anterior infarction, was discouraging.[1,2] Infarctectomy proved to be technically difficult and equally unrewarding.[3] Most surgeons retreated from intervention soon after myocardial infarction and proposed instead that the most appropriate application of bypass operations was the prevention of damage.

In the mid 1970s evidence began to accumulate that operation after infarction could be accomplished with a reasonable risk. An

ACUTE REVASCULARIZATION OF THE INFARCTED HEART   ISBN 0-8089-1870-2 important series was reported by Jones and colleagues: in 35 patients with uncontrolled pain within 30 days of infarction, coronary bypass was undertaken with no hospital mortality. Ten of these patients were operated upon within 24 hours of infarction.[4] Nunley et al reported 80 patients operated upon within 2 weeks of infarction. Mortality was 3 percent if the indication for operation was pain and 14 percent if the indication was shock.[5] These series and others demonstrated that surgical revascularization was an effective option if angina or hemodynamic instability forced early intervention after infarction.[6]

In a remarkable departure from national precedents, surgeons and cardiologists in Spokane chose to operate early (within 24 hours) upon uncomplicated as well as complicated acute infarction beginning in 1971.[7-10] Mortality in a recent report from this group was 5 percent in 440 patients with transmural infarction and 3 percent in 261 patients with a nontransmural infarction. In transmural infarction, early (less than 6 hours) revascularization was superior to later revascularization (3.8 vs. 8 percent mortality) and 3 vessel disease was a relatively high risk situation (9 percent mortality).[10] Comparison with medical treatment is difficult because the referral system in Spokane allowed several opportunities for the choice of patients especially well suited for operation.[11]

Aggressive revascularization of acute infarction also had proponents in Des Moines.[12,13] In the last ten years, patients with clinical evidence of continuing infarction (persistent chest pain or hemodynamic or electrocardiographic instability) underwent emergency catheterization. One hundred eighty-nine patients underwent immediate operation (3 percent mortality). Three hundred thirty-one patients were reperfused successfully in the catheterization laboratory (4.2 percent mortality). Seventy-two patients failed catheterization attempts at reperfusion and underwent operation (11 percent mortality). One hundred forty-six patients could not be reperfused in the catheterization laboratory and had subsequent medical treatment (17 percent mortality). Among those patients who could not be reperfused in the catheterization laboratory, patients were chosen for surgery who had evidence for potential myocardial muscle salvage as judged by endocardial anatomy and the presence of some flow to the infarcting region. These authors found no correlation between time and regional myocardial salvage, but they did find that patients with no angiographic evidence of flow to the infarcting area for 4 hours had little evidence of benefit from reperfusion.[13]

REALITIES OF EXPERIMENTAL REPERFUSION

The results of reperfusion in experimental models have done little to encourage clinical efforts at aggressive reperfusion. Jennings and colleagues, in extensive studies of circumflex coronary artery occlusion in the dog, found that occlusion for 20 minutes led to ischemia that was nearly completely reversible. After 40 minutes, 36 percent of the muscle was irreversibly damaged and after 3 hours, 90 percent of the muscle at risk was lost. Recovery of high energy phosphate stores in muscle that survived required approximately 1 week.[14]

Kloner and colleagues studied anterior descending occlusion in the dog.[15] Two hours of occlusion followed by 4 hours of reperfusion led to loss of 27 percent of the muscle, which became necrotic in the animals not reperfused. Occlusion for 3 hours led to loss of 78 percent of this muscle. Studies of functional recovery (using systolic thickening by echocardiography) revealed that after 2 hours of occlusion with 4 hours of reperfusion, there was no systolic wall thickening in the infarct zone. By 2 weeks of reperfusion, wall thickening had returned to 39 percent of normal. Permanently occluded infarcts had wall thickening that was only 3 percent of normal after 2 weeks.[15] If these animal models apply to clinical situations, reperfusion as early as 2 hours after occlusion would lead to salvage of less than 50 percent of myocardial mass and function.

Fortunately, in many clinical situations, collateral flow or limited flow through a tight stenosis allows some perfusion of the infarcting region. Phillips and colleagues found that most of the patients with favorable endocardial anatomy (i.e., patients that had a good potential for myocardial salvage from reperfusion) had some flow to the infarct area.[13] Rogers, et al studied emergency reperfusion in 63 patients with acute myocardial infarction, dividing the patients into a "no flow" group and a "limited flow" group based upon flow to the infarct area. Successful reperfusion led to an improvement in ejection fraction and in regional wall motion in the "limited flow" group while reperfusion led to no improvement in the "no flow" group. The average interval between the onset of the infarction and reperfusion in this study was approximately 8 hours. Forty-three percent of patients in this series were in the limited flow group.[16]

It is clear that clinical myocardial infarction presents to the cardiologist and surgeon a heterogeneous group of patients for whom optimal management must be individualized.

CLINICAL STRATEGIES FOR EMERGENCY SURGERY

Modification of the Operative Procedure

In patients with evolving myocardial infarction, the overwhelming consideration is rapid revascularization. We ordinarily do not wait for blood to be available. Expeditious insertion of an arterial catheter, Swan-Ganz catheter, and Foley catheter is attempted, but any of these are omitted if difficulty is encountered. The chest is opened and cardiopulmonary bypass is begun as soon as possible while saphenous veins are harvested from the legs. Local and systemic hypothermia (25°C) is used as is hyperkalemic oxygenated crystalloid cardioplegic arrest.[17] Oxygenated cardioplegic solution is infused into the area of infarction through a completed distal anastomosis. Such infusion is very difficult when the internal mammary artery has been utilized to revascularize the infarct area.[18] For this reason, and because every minute is important, internal mammary arteries are not ordinarily used. Oxygenated cardioplegic solution is reinfused into the region of infarction every 15 minutes as other distal anastomoses are completed. Proximal anastomoses are then created. After the grafts are opened, the patient remains on cardiopulmonary bypass for 20–30 minutes. Ventricular distension is carefully avoided by venting if necessary. The patient is gently weaned from cardiopulmonary bypass. Catecholamine support may be used, but if more than minimal doses of catecholamines are necessary, an intra-aortic balloon pump is considered. If the patient does not have peripheral vascular disease or small femoral arteries, we use the intra-aortic balloon pump rather than using larger doses of catecholamines.

In patients who have previously undergone coronary artery bypass grafting, expeditious surgical revascularization is more difficult. In these patients, an intra-aortic balloon pump is usually inserted at the time of catheterization and aggressive attempts are made to establish coronary flow by angioplasty techniques.

Myocardial Infarction with Known Coronary Anatomy

Occasional patients suffer infarctions or extension of infarction in the hospital after catheterization has been completed. These patients offer an excellent opportunity for rapid surgical revascularization. A recent patient illustrates this situation.

A 61-year-old female collapsed at 8:30 p.m. on the day following her catheterization. She had been scheduled for surgical revascularization the following morning. She suffered hypotension and bradycardia with ST elevation in the inferior leads on her electrocardiogram. Her catheterization had shown 80 percent diameter reduction of the left anterior descending and 95 percent narrowing of the right coronary artery. The operating room team was called in (from home) and she was transferred directly to the operating room. At 10:03 p.m. (93 minutes after the chest pain had started) oxygenated cardioplegic solution was being infused into the bypass graft to the inferior wall. She was easily weaned from cardiopulmonary bypass with no left ventricular dysfunction and moderate right ventricular dysfunction. A gated blood pool scan on the morning after operation revealed severe right ventricular dysfunction and a normal left ventricle. The gated blood pool scan was repeated 8 days later prior to discharge and revealed normal right ventricular function and normal left ventricular function with an ejection fraction of 83 percent (her preoperative angiogram had shown a hyperdynamic ventricle).

Myocardial Infarction with Unknown Coronary Anatomy

If a patient enters the hospital with an acute myocardial infarction within 4 hours of the onset of pain, he is given the option of entering a clinical trial of intravenous recombinant tissue plasminogen activator (r-TPA). If he enters the trial, a bolus of r-TPA is administered and continued as an intravenous infu-

sion. Anatomy is then defined by catheterization. After 120
minutes, other techniques (intracoronary streptokinase, angioplasty, or surgery) may be used to attempt reperfusion. If the
patient does not enter the study, he is taken directly to the
catheterization laboratory and the coronary anatomy is defined.
At this juncture, under rare circumstances, operative intervention
may be attempted without further attempts at "medical" reperfusion. These circumstances would include: (1) extremely compelling anatomy such as tight left main coronary artery stenosis or
severe triple vessel disease; (2) extreme hemodynamic instability
with power failure refractory to medical therapy including intravenous nitroglycerin, calcium antagonists, and the intra-aortic
balloon pump.

Under most circumstances, attempts would be made to medically reperfuse the area of infarction with intracoronary
streptokinase or angioplasty. After this attempt, residual coronary
stenoses would be assessed and emergency surgical intervention
reconsidered.[19-22] The following case illustrates a situation in
which emergency surgical revascularization is appropriate.

A 41-year-old male entered the hospital with unstable angina and at
2:16 p.m. had severe chest pain. Emergency cardiac catheterization
revealed a 99 percent stenosis of the left anterior descending and a 75
percent coronary artery stenosis. The patient had ventricular fibrillation
at 3:45 p.m. as the catheterization was being completed. Cardiopulmonary resuscitation was required for approximately 20 minutes and an
intra-aortic balloon pump was inserted. Anterior ST segment elevation
was present. Recurrent ventricular fibrillation that could be only temporarily reversed forced emergency operation. The bypass graft to the
anterior wall was opened at 4:45 p.m., 159 minutes after his chest pain
began. Three coronary bypass grafts were performed. His CK-MB level
peaked at 280 units postoperatively. A gated blood pool scan revealed
anterior hypokinesis with a 64 percent ejection fraction 7 days after
operation. The patient was discharged on the eighth postoperative day.

Percutaneous Transluminal Coronary Angioplasty

In skilled hands, misadventures during percutaneous transluminal coronary angioplasty (PTCA) are very rare. When they do
occur, they offer an excellent opportunity for operative salvage of
myocardium at risk.[23-27] These patients often are hemodynamically stable and can be taken quickly to the operating room

without an intra-aortic balloon pump. An excellent result is usually achieved with expeditious reperfusion. In most circumstances, patients who suffer ST segment elevation or prolonged pain with an increase in coronary artery stenosis at the time of angioplasty undergo one or two attempts at repeat angioplasty while the operating room is prepared. If severe stenosis persists, the patient is taken to the operating room. An intra-aortic balloon pump is not utilized if the operating room is immediately available. If there is to be some delay in beginning the operation or if the patient has had a previous sternotomy, an intra-aortic balloon pump is usually inserted.

A second category of patients undergoing PTCA have also undergone operation on the day of the angioplasty procedure in our institution. These are patients with compelling coronary anatomy who did not suffer ST segment elevation but had no improvement or an increase in coronary stenosis at the time of angioplasty. In these circumstances, all routine monitoring lines would be inserted preoperatively and the operation would not begin until blood is available from the blood bank.

Unstable Angina

A final subgroup of patients who have undergone emergency operation in our institution are patients with unstable angina refractory to medical therapy. Catheterization in these patients usually revealed extensive coronary disease and emergency operation was advised.[28,29]

RESULTS OF EMERGENCY OPERATION

In the 39 months from January 1983 through March 1986, 69 patients underwent emergency surgical revascularization by one of the authors (RAG). This review includes all patients undergoing coronary bypass on the day of catheterization. For the purpose of analysis, these patients are divided into patients who presented with myocardial infarction, patients who presented as failures of angioplasty, and patients who presented with unstable angina. Data are expressed as mean ± standard deviation. Results are summarized in Tables 4-1 and 4-2.

Table 4-1

Emergency Coronary Bypass Patients

	MI Group (n = 19)
Age	59.5 ± 10.4
Sex—% male	68%
Previous MI	32%
MI within 60 days	21%
CHC Angina	3.4 ± 1.1
Previous CABG	5%
Preoperative status	
Prolonged chest pain*	84%
Current of injury*	79%
Pump failure*	53%
Cardiac arrest	32%

* p < 0.01, Chi-square analysis

Table 4-2

Results of Operation

	MI Group (N = 19)
Timing of Operation (minutes)	
Operation to reperfusion	41.8 ± 30.7
Event to reperfusion	460.1 ± 500.8
Preoperative IABP*	42%
Intraoperative IABP	5%
Number of grafts performed	2.9 ± 1.0
IMA grafts*	21%
Postoperative peak CK-MB units	145.4 ± 160.1
Mortality	2(10.5%)
Postoperative day discharged	12.1 ± 10.4

[1] Significantly different (p < 0.01) from unstable angina group.

[2] Significantly different from MI group (p < 0.01) and from unstable angina group (p < 0.05).

[3] Significantly different (p < 0.01) from MI group and unstable angina group.

[4] Significantly different (p < 0.05) from MI group.

[1-4] Analysis of variance and multiple comparisons: Tukey-Kramer method[38]

* P < 0.05, Chi-square analysis.

PTCA Failure Group (n = 28)	Unstable Angina Group (n = 22)	Total Series (n = 69)
57.9 ± 10.5	57.8 ± 13.5	58.3 ± 11.4
61%	73%	67%
43%	64%	46%
25%	32%	26%
2.9 ± 1.4	3.5 ± 1.0	3.2 ± 1.2
4%	18%	9%
18%	100%	62%
57%	32%	55%
11%	14%	23%
11%	0%	13%

PTCA Failure Group (n = 28)	Unstable angina Group (n = 22)	Total series (n = 69)
33.5 ± 11.4[1]	53.9 ± 20.8	42.4 ± 22.7
144.0 ± 65.9[2]	339.5 ± 199.3	295.6 ± 306.0
7%	23%	22%
7%	0%	4%
1.8 ± 0.6[3]	3.4 ± 1.0	2.6 ± 1.1
21%	55%	32%
72.5 ± 128.3	33.8 ± 38.9[4]	80.9 ± 126.3
0	1(4.5%)	3(4.3%)
8.6 ± 2.4	8.2 ± 2.4	9.4 ± 6.0

Patients Presenting with Myocardial Infarction

Nineteen patients presented with myocardial infarction. Of these, three patients suffered infarction with known coronary anatomy. One patient, described in the example given above, suffered an acute infarction on the day following her catheterization and was taken directly to the operating room. A second patient was stable after her catheterization for several hours and then suffered a cardiac arrest with an inferior infarction. She underwent cardiopulmonary resuscitation and was taken to the operating room 135 minutes after her arrest. The third patient had an anterior infarction on the day following angioplasty. He was taken to the catheterization laboratory where the left anterior descending was found to be unsuitable for reangioplasty. He was taken to the operating room 120 minutes after infarction. All three patients had excellent results.

Eight of these 19 patients suffered an infarction, underwent catheterization, and were taken directly to the operating room. Four patients entered the emergency room with evolving myocardial infarction, two patients entered the hospital with unstable angina and suffered a myocardial infarction after admission but prior to catheterization, and two patients suffered myocardial infarctions during catheterization at other hospitals and were transferred for emergency operation.

One patient in this subgroup died after operation. This 77-year-old man underwent cardiac catheterization at another hospital on the morning of admission. His pain was treated with intravenous nitroglycerin, calcium-channel blockers, and narcotics. On admission to our hospital, he was hypotensive and in pulmonary edema. He was taken to the operating room because of power failure with an evolving anterior myocardial infarction. Revascularization was accomplished 8 hours after infarction with three bypass grafts. He remained in cardiogenic shock postoperatively despite catecholamines, vasodilators, and the intra-aortic balloon pump. He died 20 days after operation.

Eight patients presented with myocardial infarction and underwent an attempt at medical revascularization prior to operation. Four patients presented to the emergency room with infarction, two patients entered the hospital with unstable angina, and two patients suffered infarction after successful angioplasty. Of these eight patients, seven were given intracoronary or intravenous thrombolytic agents and five patients underwent angio-plasty.

There was one death in this subgroup. A 43-year-old female entered the hospital 50 minutes after an anterior infarction. She suffered occlu-sion of the circumflex artery during infusion of intracoronary streptokinase. Her left anterior descending and circumflex were therefore both temporarily occluded. After further treatment with intracoronary streptokinase, the vessels were reopened. Because of residual stenosis, she was taken to the operating room after three hours in the catheteriza-tion laboratory. Postoperatively, she required catecholamines and the intra-aortic balloon pump. She developed noncardiogenic pulmonary edema and subsequent sepsis and died 7 days after operation.

Considering all 19 patients who presented with myocardial infarction, the mean time from infarction to coronary reperfusion was 460 ± 501 minutes with a median of 309 minutes. The mean peak CK-MB isoenzyme level postoperatively was 145 ± 160 units. There were two deaths in this group. The indications for emergency operation were chest pain in 84 percent, ST segment elevation in 79 percent, power failure (hypotension requiring catecholamine infusion or LVEDP greater than 30 mmHg or acute pulmonary edema) in 53 percent, and cardiac arrest in 32 percent. The average postoperative hospital stay was 12.1 ± 10.4 days.

Failures of Percutaneous Transluminal Coronary Angioplasty

In the 39 months under consideration, 17 patients suffered a myocardial infarction requiring emergency operation while un-dergoing PTCA. Eleven additional patients underwent PTCA followed by urgent coronary bypass without a definite infarction. Of these 11 patients, 5 suffered coronary dissection without coronary occlusion, 3 had dissection with coronary occlusion, 2 patients with double vessel disease underwent unsuccessful angioplasty without dissection or occlusion, and 1 patient with single vessel disease (multiple lesions in the left anterior descend-ing) could not be dilated.

In the 28 patients who had emergency operation after failed angioplasty, 18 percent had prolonged chest pain, 57 percent had ST segment elevation, 11 percent had power failure, and 11 percent suffered cardiac arrest. The mean time to reperfusion was 144 ± 66 minutes with a median time of 138 minutes. The peak CK-MB level was 72 ± 128 units. There were no deaths in this subgroup. The average postoperative hospitalization was 8.6 ± 2.3 days.

Unstable Angina

Twenty-two patients presented with unstable angina. The most common reason for emergency operation in this subgroup was compelling coronary anatomy. Five patients had severe left main coronary artery stenosis (4 of these were combined with greater than 90 percent stenosis of the right coronary artery). Eleven patients had severe triple vessel coronary disease including greater than 90 percent stenosis of the left anterior descending. Sixty-four percent of these patients had had previous myocardial infarctions and 31 percent had unstable angina after a recent infarction.

The indications for operation in this subgroup were chest pain—100 percent, ST segment elevation—32 percent, power failure—14 percent, and cardiac arrest—0. The mean time to reperfusion was 340 ± 199 minutes (after catheterization) with a median time of 360 minutes. The mean peak postoperative CK-MB level was 34 ± 39 units. The average hospital stay after operation was 8.2 ± 2.4 days. There was one death in this subgroup.

A 78-year-old obese female with renal failure presented with unstable angina 3 days after an inferior infarction. Catheterization revealed total occlusion of the left anterior descending, total occlusion of the right coronary artery, 90 percent stenosis of the circumflex, an ejection fraction of 29 percent, and a left ventricular end diastolic pressure of 36 mmHg. The patient had power failure with pulmonary edema preoperatively. After operation, she had profound power failure and died one day later.

Postoperative Complications

The incidence of complications after operation was not different in the various groups. In the total series, 62 percent required inotropic support, 32 percent were treated for postoperative arrhythmias, 22 percent were treated for postoperative pericarditis, and 4 percent had positive blood cultures. There were no mediastinal wound problems and no patient had cardiac tamponade.

DISCUSSION

Analysis of Results

This retrospective review emphasizes the disparity between clinical plans and the realities of clinical care. This was especially evident in analysis of the time between pain and revascularization. We plan completion of emergency surgical revascularization within 3 hours of pain onset, but this was accomplished only in patients after failed PTCA. In the myocardial infarction subgroup, transfer from other hospitals, delay prior to catheterization, and attempted medical reperfusion led to a median time of 5 hours from pain to reperfusion. The mean time prior to reperfusion was extended to 7⅔ hours by one patient whose pain began 38 hours before revascularization. In patients with PTCA failure, the decision to operate was occasionally delayed by further attempts to reopen a closed vessel. These attempts were often successful and prevented operation. On other occasions, the artery could be temporarily reopened until the operating room was ready. The average time between the precipitating event and revascularization was 144 minutes (67 minutes in the catheterization laboratory, 42 minutes in the operating room prior to skin incision, and 35 minutes after incision before infusion of an oxygenated solution into the ischemic region). The shortest time between event and reperfusion was 90 minutes in the MI group and 55 minutes in the PTCA group. When this shortest time is compared to the average time, the disparity between planning and execution is sobering. This reality is not unique to our series: The mean time to revascularization was 6⅓ hours in Berg's series from Spokane,[9] which did not include any patients more than 12 hours after infarction, and 8 hours in Phillips' series from Des Moines.[12]

Analysis of the MI group reveals that operation was usually accomplished for complicated infarction, not for uncomplicated infarction. Fifty-three percent of this group had power failure, 32 percent had a cardiac arrest, and 42 percent had an intra-aortic balloom pump placed preoperatively. All of these patients had elevation of postoperative peak CK-MB levels, with an average level twice that found in the PTCA group and four times that found in the unstable angina group.

The PTCA group contained 17 patients with definite evidence of infarction prior to operation. We have not followed the suggestion made by Murphy, et al that an intra-aortic balloon pump might be used in these patients.[23] Indeed, only two patients were treated in this manner. If an operating room is immediately available, we believe that expeditious revascularization is more important than delaying for insertion of the assist device. There was no mortality in our PTCA group, but these results do not necessarily support our limited use of the balloon pump.

Eleven patients in the PTCA group did not have definite evidence of infarction prior to operation. Eight of these patients had coronary dissection with or without occlusion and the stenosis could not be crossed in the other three patients. Several of these patients had ST segment elevation but it did not persist as the patient was taken to the operating room. Results were excellent in this subgroup, with low peak postoperative CK-MB isoenzyme levels (25 ± 25 units) and no mortality.

The unstable angina group represents a group of patients with a compelling pain pattern combined with compelling coronary pathology. Thirty-two percent of these patients had at least transient ST elevation preoperatively, but there was no evolution of infarction by electrocardiogram. Twenty-three percent of this group required an intra-aortic balloon pump prior to operation. CK-MB levels were low, but were more than twice as high as the level achieved in this hospital in elective operations.[17,18]

Revascularization was accomplished primarily with vein grafts both for speed and for ease of cardioplegia infusion into the area of severe ischemia.[18] Of the 36 patients with definite preoperative infarction, 6 had internal mammary grafts (17 percent), while 16 of the 33 patients without infarction had mammary grafts (48 percent).

Mortality in 2 of the 3 deaths in this series was directly related to severe preoperative pump failure in elderly (age greater than 75) patients. Perhaps, as suggested by Cohn, the elderly patients should be treated differently.[30] In this series, 2 of 7 patients older than 75 died (29 percent) while only 1 of 62 patients less than 76 died (1.6 percent). The third death occurred in a young patient who suffered a complication of medical reperfusion with circumflex occlusion during attempted infusion of streptokinase into the left anterior descending artery. She survived the operation with reasonable hemodynamic function, but developed noncardiogenic pulmonary edema, subsequent pulmonary infection, and septic shock. This single death in a young patient must be considered in light of the experience of Phillips et al. In their series, immediate surgical reperfusion had a 3 percent mortality while surgical reperfusion after attempted medical reperfusion led to an 11 percent mortality.[13] One would certainly expect that a prolonged attempt at medical reperfusion would increase the risk of subsequent operation.

Complications after operation were unusual in this series. The mean hopsitalization after operation was only 9.4 ± 6.0 days. Emergency operation has been an effective therapeutic option in our institution with a low mortality (1.6 percent) in patients under the age of 76.

Current Strategy for Reperfusion

Early thrombolysis appears to be the best hope for muscle salvage early after infarction. Trials of intravenous and intracoronary streptokinase have generally been disappointing, although some large studies have shown significant benefit if the drug can be given early after the onset of ischemia.[31-34] Recombinant tissue plasminogen activator, on the other hand, appears to be more effective in opening occluded coronary vessels.[35-37] A high incidence of reclosure has encouraged the early use of PTCA or surgical revascularization.[22,35,37]

Our current policy is enrollment of consenting acute (less than 4 hours) infarction patients (under the age of 70 with certain medical restrictions) in a study of intravenous r-TPA. A control group of patients receives intracoronary streptokinase. Coronary angiography is performed 60 minutes, 90 minutes, and 120 minutes after r-TPA or streptokinase infusion is begun. After 120 minutes, residual stenosis is treated with angioplasty if feasible. Only the vessel perfusing the area of infarction is dilated. A critical consideration is the presence of pump failure during occlusion of the target artery. If pump failure was present prior to thrombolysis, then angioplasty may lead to reocclusion and renewed pump failure. In this circumstance, close surgical backup is confirmed and consideration is given to emergency operation if the angioplasty is difficult. If no pump failure was present prior to thrombolysis, angioplasty may proceed with little risk of acute hemodynamic decompensation, even if there is significant disease in coronaries other than the target vessel.

In 6 months, 26 patients have been enrolled in this study. Reperfusion was accomplished in 18 of 21 patients who received r-TPA and in 1 of 5 patients who received streptokinase. Emergency operation was necessary in only two patients and elective operation was accomplished in three additional patients. There have been no deaths and one major complication (subdural hematoma requiring evacuation).

Our strategy generally reserves early operative intervention for patients with complicated infarction, that is, threatened power failure or threatened extension of the original infarct (persistence or recurrence of pain or ECG changes). Our experience has shown emergency operation to be a very effective therapeutic option in these high risk circumstances and we do not hesitate to use it, even in the first few hours after infarction.

In most patients with uncomplicated myocardial infarction, presentation to the hospital is delayed and surgical revascularization cannot be accomplished before 5 or 6 hours after the onset of pain. In this situation, coronary bypass for muscle salvage is not attempted. There are unusual instances, however, in which surgical revascularization can be accomplished within three hours, such as infarction during PTCA or infarction in the hospital with known anatomy. In these circumstances, emergency operation may salvage myocardium and we proceed immediately.

Emergency surgical revascularization is a safe and effective therapeutic option. Myocardial infarction, however, is a heterogeneous disease and surgical revascularization should be intelligently combined on a patient-by-patient basis with other techniques of coronary revascularization.

REFERENCES

1. Leinbach RC, Gold HK, Dinsmore RE, et al: The role of angiography in cardiogenic shock. Circulation 47/48(Suppl II): II-95–II-98, 1973
2. Mundth ED, Buckley MJ, Leinbach RC, et al: Surgical intervention

for the complications of acute myocardial ischemia. Ann Surg 178:379–390, 1973

3. Daggett WM, Buckley MJ, Mundth ED, et al: The role of infarctectomy in the surgical treatment of myocardial infarction. Am Heart J 84:723–726, 1972

4. Jones EL, Douglas JS, Jr., Craver JM, et al: Results of coronary revascularization in patients with recent myocardial infarction. J Thorac Cardiovasc Surg 76:545–551, 1978

5. Nunley DL, Grunkemeier GL, Teply JF, et al: Coronary bypass operation following acute complicated myocardial infarction. J Thorac Cardiovasc Surg 85:485–491, 1983

6. Fudge TL, Harrington OB, Crosby VG, et al: Coronary artery bypass after recent myocardial infarction. Arch Surg 117:1418–1420, 1982

7. Berg R, Jr., Selinger SL, Leonard JJ, et al: Immediate coronary artery bypass for acute evolving infarction. J Thorac Cardiovasc Surg 81:492–497, 1981

8. Selinger SL, Berg R, Jr., Leonard JJ, et al: Surgical treatment of acute evolving anterior myocardial infarction. Circulation 64(Suppl II):II-28–II-33, 1981

9. Berg R, Jr., Selinger SL, Leonard JJ, et al: Acute evolving myocardial infarction: a surgical emergency. J Thorac Cardiovasc Surg 88: 902–906, 1984

10. DeWood MA, Spores J, Berg R, Jr., et al: Acute myocardial infarction: a decade of experience with surgical reperfusion in 701 patients. Circulation 68(Suppl II):II-8–II-16, 1983

11. Spencer FC: Emergency coronary bypass for acute infarction: an unproved clinical experiment. Circulation 68(Suppl II):II-17–II-19, 1983

12. Phillips SJ, Kongtahworn C, Skinner JR, et al: Emergency coronary artery reperfusion: a choice therapy for evolving myocardial infarction. J Thorac Cardiovasc Surg 86:679–688, 1983

13. Phillips SJ, Zeff RH, Skinner JR, et al: Reperfusion protocol and results in 738 patients with evolving myocardial infarction. Ann Thorac Surg 41:119–124, 1986

14. Jennings RB, Reimer KA: Factors involved in salvaging ischemic myocardium: Effect of reperfusion of arterial blood. Circulation 68(Suppl I):I-25–I-36, 1983

15. Kloner RA, Ellis SG, Lange R, et al: Studies of experimental coronary artery reperfusion: Effects on infarct size, myocardial function, biochemistry, ultrastructure and microvascular damage. Circulation 68 (Suppl I):I-8–I-15, 1983

16. Rogers WJ, Hood WP, Jr., Mantle JA, et al: Return of left ventricular function after reperfusion in patients with myocardial infarction:

importance of subtotal stenoses or intact collaterals. Circulation 69:338–349, 1984

17. Guyton RA, Dorsey LMA, Craver JM, et al: Improved myocardial recovery after cardioplegic arrest with an oxygenated crystalloid solution. J Thorac Cardiovasc Surg 89:877–887, 1985

18. Guyton RA, Craver JM, Hatcher CR, Jr.: Myocardial protection with oxygenated crystalloid cardioplegia for internal mammary artery bypass grafting. Presented at Southern Thoracic Surgical Association, Hilton Head, SC, November 1, 1984

19. Messmer BJ, Merx W, Meyer J, et al: New developments in medical-surgical treatment of myocardial infarction. Ann Thorac Surg 35:70–79, 1983

20. Skinner JR, Phillips SJ, Zeff RH, et al: Immediate coronary bypass following failed streptokinase infusion in evolving myocardial infarction. J Thorac Cardiovasc Surg 87:567–570, 1984

21. Kay P, Ahmad A, Floten S, et al: Emergency coronary artery bypass surgery after intracoronary thrombolysis for evolving myocardial infarction. Br Heart J 53:260–264, 1985

22. Anderson JL, Battistessa SA, Clayton PD, et al: Coronary bypass surgery early after thrombolytic therapy for acute myocardial infarction. Ann Thorac Surg 41:176–183, 1986

23. Murphy DA, Craver JM, Jones EL, et al: Surgical revascularization following unsuccessful percutaneous transluminal coronary angioplasty. J Thorac Cardiovasc Surg 84:342–348, 1982

24. Cowley MJ, Dorros G, Kelsey SF, et al: Emergency coronary bypass surgery after coronary angioplasty: the National Heart, Lung, and Blood Institute's percutaneous transluminal coronary angioplasty registry experience. Am J Cardiol 53:22C–26C, 1984

25. Killen DA, Hamaker WR, Reed WA: Coronary artery bypass following percutaneous transluminal coronary angioplasty. Ann Thorac Surg 40:133–138, 1985

26. Brahos GJ, Baker NH, Ewy HG, et al: Aortocoronary bypass following unsuccessful PTCA: experience in 100 consecutive patients. Ann Thorac Surg 40:7–10, 1985

27. Pelletier LC, Pardini A, Renkin J, et al: Myocardial revascularization after failure of percutaneous transluminal coronary angioplasty. J Thorac Cardiovasc Surg 90:265–271, 1985

28. Rahimtoola SH: Coronary bypass surgery for unstable angina. Circulation 69:842–848, 1984

29. Jones EL, Waites TF, Craver JM, et al: Unstable angina pectoris: comparison with the National Cooperative Study. Ann Thorac Surg 34:427–434, 1982

30. Cohn LH: In discussion of Reperfusion protocol and results in 738

patients with evolving myocardial infarction. Ann Thorac Surg 41:119–124, 1986

31. Hillis LD, Borer J, Braunwald E, et al: High dose intravenous streptokinase for acute myocardial infarction: preliminary results of a multicenter trial. J Am Coll Cardiol 6:957–962, 1985

32. Serruys PW, Simoons ML, Suryapranata H, et al: Preservation of global and regional left ventricular function after early thrombolysis in acute myocardial infarction. J Am Coll Cardiol 7:729–742, 1986

33. The Trial of the Italian Group for the Study of Streptokinase in Myocardial Infarction: Effectiveness of intravenous thrombolytic treatment in acute myocardial infarctions. Lancet Feb 22:397–401, 1986

34. Mathey DG, Sheehan FH, Schofer J, et al: Time from onset of symptoms to thrombolytic therapy: a major determinant of myocardial salvage in patients with acute transmural infarction. J Am Coll Cardiol 6:518–525, 1985

35. Gold HK, Leinbach RC, Garabedian HD, et al: Acute coronary reocclusion after thrombolysis with recominant human tissue-type plasminogen activator: prevention by a maintenance infusion. Circulation 73:347–352, 1986

36. Williams DO, Borer J, Braunwald E, et al: Intravenous recombinant tissue-type plasminogen activator in patients with acute myocardial infarction: a report from the NHLBI thrombolysis in myocardial infarction trail. Circulation 73:338–346, 1986

37. Topol EJ, Weiss JL, Brinker JA, et al: Regional wall motion improvement after coronary thrombolysis with recombinant tissue plasminogen activator: importance of coronary angioplasty. J Am Coll Cardiol 6:426–433, 1985

38. Kramer CY: Extension of multiple range tests to group means with unequal numbers. Biometrics 12:307–310, 1956

Index

Page numbers in *italics*
indicate illustrations.

Acute myocardial infarction
    (AMI)
  coronary artery bypass
    grafting, and elective
    CABG, comparison of,
    49–54
  management of, using
    emergency
    angioplasty, 17–33
  percutaneous transluminal
    coronary angioplasty
    during, 22–32. *See
    also* Percutaneous
    transluminal coronary
    angioplasty (PTCA)
  reperfusion of. *See*
    Reperfusion of acute
    myocardial infarction
  salvage of. *See* Salvage of
    acute myocardial
    infarction
  surgical management of, 85–
    80. *See also* Surgical
    management of acute
    myocardial infarction
Anesthesia
  for emergency coronary
    artery bypass grafting,

48–54. *See also*
    Coronary artery
    bypass grafting
    (CABG)
  for nonsurgical myocardial
    reperfusion, 54–58
  in reperfusion of acute
    myocardial infarction,
    35–58
Anesthetics
  effect of, on ischemic
    myocardium, 36–48
  inhalation, ischemic
    myocardium and, 36–
    44
  intravenous, ischemic
    myocardium and, 44–
    47
  regional, ischemic
    myocardium and, 48
Angina, unstable, emergency
    surgery for acute
    myocardial infarction
    in, 71
  results of, 76
Angioplasty
  coronary, percutaneous
    transluminal
  emergency
    for acute myocardial
    infarction, 70–71
    Duke experience using,

Angioplasty (*continued*)
        22–32. *See also*
        Percutaneous
        transluminal coronary
        angioplasty (PTCA)
    and streptokinase for
        reperfusion,
        anesthesia for, 54–58
    emergency, in acute
        myocardial infarction
        management, 17–33

Bezoid-Jarish reflexes,
        stimulation of, by
        reperfusion, 10
Blood flow
    coronary, intravenous
        anesthetics and, 45
    myocardial, inhalation
        anesthetics and, 42

Cardioinhibitory
        vasodepressor
        reflexes, stimulation
        of, reperfusion, 10
Catecholamine levels,
        inhalation anesthetics
        and, in acute
        myocardial infarction,
        36–39
Catheterization, cardiac,
        interventional
        program of, 22–32.
        See also Percutaneous
        transluminal coronary
        angioplasty (PTCA)
Coronary artery bypass
        grafting (CABG), 48–
        54
    for AMI and elective
        patients, comparison
        of, 49–54

Coronary artery disease,
        collaterized
        myocardial
        circulation in
        response to, 7–8

Diazepam, ischemic
        myocardium and, 46,
        47
Dogs, collateralized
        myocardial
        circulation in, 6–7

Ejection fraction, global, after
        reperfusion, 19–21
Englurane, myocardial blood
        flow and, 42
Epidural anesthesia, ischemic
        myocardium and, 48
Etomidate, ischemic
        myocardium and, 46–
        47

Fentanyl, ischemic
        myocardium and, 46,
        47

Halothane
    effect of, on ischemic
        myocardial tissue,
        43–44, 45
    ischemic myocardium and,
        40
    myocardial blood flow and,
        42
Humans, collaterized
        myocardial
        circulation in, 7–8

Infarction, extent of,
        determination of, 3
Inhalation anesthetics,

ischemic myocardium
and, 36–44
Interventional cardiac
catheterization
program, 22–32. See
also Percutaneous
transluminal coronary
angioplasty (PTCA)
Intravenous anesthetics,
ischemic myocardium
and, 44–47
Ischemic myocardium, effect
of anesthetic drugs
on, 36–48
Isoflurane, coronary vascular
effect of, 42

Ketamine, ischemic
myocardium and, 44–
46

Midazolam, ischemic
myocardium and, 46,
47
Myocardium
acutely infarcted,
reperfusion of. See
Reperfusion of acute
myocardial infarction
ischemic, effect of anesthetic
drugs on, 36–48

Oxygen consumption,
myocardial
inhalation anesthetics and,
39–41
intravenous anesthetics and,
45
regional anesthesia and, 48

Percutaneous transluminal
coronary angioplasty

(PTCA)
with adjunctive
thrombolytic therapy
vs. streptokinase
alone, 31–32
emergency
in acute myocardial
infarction, 70–71
failures of, 75–76
Duke experience using,
22–32
methods of, 24–28
patient selected for, 24
results of, 29–30
and streptokinase for
reperfusion,
anesthesia for, 54–58
Pigs, collateralized myocardial
circulation in, 7

Reflexes, vasodepressor,
cardioinhibitory,
stimulation of, by
reperfusion, 10
Regional anesthesia, ischemic
myocardium and, 48
anesthesia in, 35–58
clinical studies of, 18–22
current strategy for, 79–80
differences in methodology
versus outcome of,
10–11
emergency surgical,
anesthetic
management of, 48–
54. See also Coronary
artery bypass grafting
(CABG)
experimental, realities of,
67–68
factors possibly determining
outcome/advisability

Reperfusion of myocardial
        infarction (continued)
        of, 8–10
    nonsurgical, anesthesia
        management for, 54–
        58
    scientific foundations for, 1–
        11
    time limit for, 2

Salvage of acute myocardial
        infarction
    debate over, 5–6
    decision on, 2–6
    early thrombolysis for, 79–
        80
    experimental studies of, 17–
        18
    functional consequences of,
        4–5
    limitations on, 22
Spinal anesthesia, ischemic
        myocardium and, 48
Stenosis, residual, after
        reperfusion, 9, 22
Streptokinase therapy
    early, for salvage after
        infarction, 79–80
    in reperfusion,
        complications of, 53–
        54
    vs. PTCA and adjunctive
        thrombolytic therapy,
        31–32
Surgical management of acute
        myocardial infarction,
        65–80
    emergency
        clinical strategies for, 68–
            80
        complications of, 76
        with known coronary

anatomy, 69
    modification operative
        procedure for, 68–69
    percutaneous transluminal
        coronary angioplasty
        in, 70–71
    results of, 71–76
        analysis of, 77–79
        failures of PTCA in, 75–
            76
        in patients presenting
            with myocardial
            infarction, 74–75
        in unstable angina, 76
        with unknown coronary
            anatomy, 69–70
    in unstable angina, 71
    experimental reperfusion in,
        realities of, 67–68
    historical perspective on,
        65–67

Thiopental, ischemic
        myocardium and, 44–
        46
Thrombolysis, early, for
        salvage after
        infarction, 79–80

Unstable angina, emergency
        surgery for acute
        myocardial infarction
        in, 71
    results of, 76

Vasodepressor reflexes,
        cardioinhibitory,
        stimulation of, by
        reperfusion, 10
Ventricular wall motion after
        reperfusion, 19–21
    timing and, 9–10